"This book is a uniquely successful guide towards a deeper understanding of both the reader's own body dynamics as well as yoga in its fuller context. The book addresses the physical and emotional consequences of living with scoliosis through therapeutic poses, breathing techniques, and intention-setting that the reader can easily adopt at home. I highly recommend this book to both patients and clinicians alike."

—*Melanie R. Fiorella, MD, Center for Integrative Medicine, UC San Diego Health*

# Scoliosis,
# Yoga Therapy,

*and the Art of Letting Go*

# Scoliosis, Yoga Therapy,
## *and the Art of Letting Go*

**RACHEL KRENTZMAN PT, E-RYT**
**Foreword by Matthew J. Taylor PT, PhD**

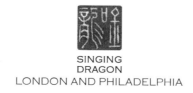

SINGING
DRAGON
LONDON AND PHILADELPHIA

First published in 2017
by Singing Dragon
an imprint of Jessica Kingsley Publishers
73 Collier Street
London N1 9BE, UK
and
400 Market Street, Suite 400
Philadelphia, PA 19106, USA

*www.singingdragon.com*

Copyright © Rachel Krentzman 2017
Foreword copyright © Matthew J. Taylor 2017
Photographs copyright © Tim Hardy 2017
*shotbyhardy.com*
Illustrations copyright © Lior Hikrey 2017

Front cover image source: Tim Hardy. The cover image is for illustrative
purposes only, and any person featuring is a model.

Cover model: Shawnee Thornton Hardy
Interior models: Aman Keays, Shawnee Thornton Hardy, Anne Marie Welsh and Rachel Krentzman

**Library of Congress Cataloging in Publication Data**
Names: Krentzman, Rachel, author.
Title: Scoliosis, yoga therapy, and the art of letting go / Rachel Krentzman
   ; foreword by Matthew J. Taylor.
Description: London ; Philadelphia : Jessica Kingsley Publishers, 2017. |
   Includes bibliographical references.
Identifiers: LCCN 2016011811 | ISBN 9781848192720
Subjects: LCSH: Scoliosis--Popular works. | Spine--Abnormalities--Popular
   works. | Yoga--Therapeutic use--Popular works.
Classification: LCC RD771.S3 K74 2017 | DDC 616.7/3--dc23 LC
record available at https://lccn.loc.gov/2016011811

**British Library Cataloguing in Publication Data**
A CIP catalogue record for this book is available from the British Library

ISBN 978 1 84819 272 0
eISBN 978 0 85701 243 2

Printed and bound in the United States

# Contents

# Foreword

I met Rachel Krentzman the first week of November 2001 at my seminar on yoga in rehabilitation in New York City. Air traffic was just settling into its new routine, so I wondered who would still make the trip so shortly after 9/11? I saw Rachel's name on the attendee list and noted her home address in California. What kind of a "nut," I wondered, would fly into NYC for this seminar? Turns out that nut was an acorn. She was pulled from within by something far stronger than the fear outside her.

Today Rachel is a strong, nurturing oak. Her gift of *Scoliosis, Yoga Therapy, and the Art of Letting Go* is her second book to bring the healing power of yoga to our twisted and contorted world. So often, caring for scoliosis has involved a forceful, external struggle against perceived deformity. Krentzman will have none of that!

Instead she invites you, the reader, to move from a fiery "struggle against" into the refreshing shade of "being with" one's curves. Yes, the book is chock-full of smart, safe, and appropriate things to do to explore and work with your curves; but, in the end, a deep silent force makes her approach different. Her invitation to sense and experience your inner qualities and wisdom gently supports the entire book.

The image of an arborist staking and pulling at the trunk and branches of a tree is commonly employed in scoliosis care. That visual reveals our society's penchant for manipulating and forcing change on others and ourselves. Rachel calls you to explore with the same sagacity that a true craftsman among arborists brings to his task. The craftsman knows that, while outer support and lines of tension can aid the process of developing the tree to its potential, more important things actually determine the vigor, vitality, and longevity of the tree. The craftsman arborist works with the tree's inner nature, its quiet drive to flourish, and describes forces that include water pressure in the cells, the genetic inclination towards full potency for its species' survival, and its biomechanical dance with gravity for optimal growth.

Like a wise and healing craftswoman, Rachel invites you to discover those same types of quiet powers within yourself and in your graceful curves. We humans have a heart–mind energy that whispers our deepest yearnings. Only when that force is also tended can the internal stability that creates presence, passion, and compassion flow like sap nourishing the tree of your spine, and life. She offers many simple, but important, tools for discovering and nurturing the inner powers so critical for you to find true fulfillment in the world.

Rachel also knows too well that the tiny, supported tree doesn't grow in isolation. She encourages you also to utilize your human equivalents of sunlight, soil, and roots. In an age during which most yoga books focus on actions, Rachel asks you not to stop there. Instead she guides you to explore yoga's wise and ancient precepts for living well: the yamas and the niyamas. Without knowing towards what light are you being pulled, how can you thrive? If you fail to tend to your roots—those origins you hold most dear and from which you grow your life—how can strength and longevity unfold? By rooting yourself in the yamas and niyamas, you can begin to be nourished by the interconnected roots of your support community. You can move towards the bright light of mystery that stirs the seed to sprout, the leaf to unfurl, and the flower to bloom.

Rachel's instructions and her personal examples will bring you to what she knows is the taproot of your being: the final niyama, which she calls "the art of letting go." Surrendering and letting go creates the possibility of reaching up and out. Paradoxically, as in a Zen koan, the one requires the other. Rachel invites you and instructs you how to fall gracefully into the mysteries of your life so you can bring forth your one, unique, and oh so important way of being in the world with all the perfection of the imperfection of every mighty tree. She shows you that it is only in your personal practice of tending, nurturing, and guiding yourself that you—or any of us—can ever hope to mend and straighten our larger world from the twists and turns of hatred and fear.

Grab your gardening gloves and boots. Under her wise direction, we all have work to do.

*Matthew J. Taylor PT, PhD*
*Former President, International*
*Association of Yoga Therapists*
*March 2016*

# Introduction

*You can't cross the sea merely by standing and staring at the water.*
**RABINDRANATH TAGORE**

Swimming in the open water has always given me a sense of peace and provided solace for me when life on land seemed confusing and difficult. Somehow diving beneath the surface and allowing the temporary silence to wash over me is my way of quieting the noise in my mind enough to feel supported by the flow of life. It reminds me of what I strive for in my yoga and meditation practice, a feeling that everything is as it should be, perfectly imperfect and unfolding in its own time.

I am learning that the key to swimming long distances in the open water is finding a way to exert the least effort possible so that I can glide calmly through the water at a good pace and avoid tiring. Every little modification of technique can dramatically change the way I am using my body and can make all the difference between a very pleasurable or an extremely exhausting swim. During my 20 years as a physical therapist and 15 years as a yoga therapist and instructor, I am seeing more and more that this is really a metaphor for how to approach not only back pain, but life in general. We often struggle and fight against the current only to find ourselves exhausted and right back where we started.

I believe that this illustration holds the key to treating scoliosis. From working with clients over the years with varying degrees of curvature, I have noticed that treatment approaches are mostly aimed at reversing the curve by applying pressure in the opposite direction with a brace or by eliminating movement altogether with surgery.

In both cases, we are working *against* the current and trying to force the curve to move in the opposite direction. My clients who have worn a brace in their teenaged years often come to me with hypersensitivity to touch and decreased body awareness because of the constant pressure of the brace on their curves. While the brace may have, at best, prevented progression of the scoliosis, it also created a great deal of muscular tension and rigidity. In addition, these clients never received any guidance or instruction for physical exercises to help their condition, so they have little connection to their body's needs and little awareness of how their spines function. They are virtually at a loss about how to manage their condition, let alone actually improve their curves.

I believe Purna Yoga therapy provides alternative solutions aimed at allowing the body to transform naturally. In looking at the physical body as an integrated and organic structure, we can provide tools that encourage a process of "letting go," along with functional re-alignment that is not invasive or aggressive. This may require a shift in perspective of what a "normal" spine should look like and it will most certainly require effort and commitment. *But if we provide the right conditions, perhaps the spine can unwind from the inside out.* In modern medicine, we sometimes look outside ourselves for solutions, forgetting that the best healer is our own body and mind.

When I was 16, my pediatrician diagnosed me with scoliosis and just told me to "keep an eye on it." Although it was a mild case, I still found that over the years it impacted me through chronic muscle tension and limited mobility in sports. Only when I started to practice Purna Yoga regularly did the pain disappear, but new problems continued to arise as I worked my way into more advanced postures. I believe that those with scoliosis benefit a great deal from yoga and should practice regularly, but with attention to what serves their bodies best. Not every style of yoga, nor every pose, is suited for each body, each spine, and each unique curve. It is important to know the ideal way to work with your spine; this requires an understanding of how to work with scoliosis itself. Transformation begins and ends with self-awareness, which is both a prerequisite and the aim of a solid and regular yoga practice.

In the pages that follow, we will explore and learn more about what scoliosis is, what yoga therapy is, and how you can begin to practice with the aim of normalizing the curve of your spine and/or preventing it from getting worse. These tools can be practiced by anyone, at any age, to find relief from muscular tension, pain, and limited mobility. It is my hope that this guide gives those of you with scoliosis the tools to get started on a path towards self-care so that you can enjoy a vibrant, active, and pain-free existence. But even more so, that you can live in peace and harmony with the twists and turns in your bodies and your lives.

*Rachel Krentzman PT, E-RYT*
*Ra'anana, Israel*
*October 2015*

# The Principles
## PART I

# CHAPTER 1

# Understanding Scoliosis

To work well with scoliosis, as with any challenge in your body, an attitude of softening can be the most helpful approach to the condition. Instead of trying to "fight" the curve by twisting it and manipulating it in the opposite direction, perhaps a little more kindness will yield better results. Consider what happens when you try to pull a toy out of a dog's mouth. He pulls harder to counter the force. And what happens when you distract the dog instead by encouraging him to focus on something else? He will loosen his grip and simply let go. In working with back pain over the years I have learned that this is a better approach towards healing. What if we became experts at letting go? If we allow the body to let go of its hold on itself, the spine might unwind and find its own balance. Do we really need to control everything to the point where we manipulate ourselves or others? Is there another way? In mindfulness-based therapy, we don't try to force ourselves to change, we learn to listen to our bodies. We observe, we feel, we let things be. In that awareness lies the key to healing. Shouldn't this principle apply to the body as well?

Listening is a skill; letting go, an even harder skill. And before we can even practice those seemingly easy concepts, we need to back them up with a little knowledge.

Consider the story of Danielle. At 19, she came to me through the encouragement of her mother who was a yoga student of mine. Danielle had a significant scoliotic curve that was impacting her life on a daily basis. She had worn a brace throughout her teenaged years, yet she still had limited range of motion in her shoulders that prevented her from lifting her arms overhead. She also experienced chronic back pain and tension. She had no body awareness and could not stand still for a minute. Her head tilted to the side. She was unaware of how to isolate different movements, and she quickly became impatient with breathing and holding still. When I touched or massaged around her spinal curve, her muscles would instinctively go into spasm, as if they were fighting back against a threat. She said that wearing the brace for four years was extremely uncomfortable for her, and that her body had always been sensitive since she took the brace off. She saw the brace as an outside force, aggressive and painful. Her body was used to fighting it at every turn.

We began with simple exercises to increase Danielle's body awareness and focus. These included postural exercises, such as Tadasana (mountain pose), as well as hip openers to help free up the pelvis and increase awareness of the connection between the pelvis and the rest of the spine. We worked together on learning how to breathe in supported positions to lessen the curve, and only then introduced traction slowly and methodically to teach the muscles to let go. I was careful not to touch her around the curve initially, as touch still led to spasm and she could not handle it. My focus was just on trying to get her to be more embodied. Strength and discipline became big parts of her treatment, and we worked on getting in touch with core muscles and not giving up during difficult exercises. I encouraged Danielle to stay in Savasana (corpse pose) for longer than she was comfortable with, with appropriate support to normalize the curve. To be honest, I was skeptical at best, and uncertain of whether she would see—or feel—the benefits. Somehow, she kept coming back, even though she was unable to remain fully present during the sessions.

After a year and a half, a moment came in which things really "clicked." Suddenly, she was excited about treatment and felt proud of her body. She began to practice acceptance and naturally felt more joy in her life. This led to her decision to commit even more to her practice out of self-love. She began to let me touch the curve. Like a little child who was beginning to trust a stranger, she allowed her muscles to soften as I massaged the areas of tightness and tension. Hanging on the yoga wall to create length and space in her spine became Danielle's favorite part of treatment.

While most physicians tend to recommend a "wait and see" approach to scoliosis, this attitude often leaves young people and their parents with a huge question mark about whether they can prevent the curve from worsening instead of simply waiting for surgery. Conservative treatment tends to favor the use of braces and/or scoliosis-specific physiotherapeutic exercises that have been shown to be beneficial in a recent overview of such exercises by Zaina *et al.* (2015). Still, the research remains limited in this area because of difficulty with designing ethical studies and the need for long-term follow up.

Dr. Loren Fishman, a physiatrist and yoga practitioner in New York, and his colleagues published the first study (2014) on the benefits of yoga for scoliosis. They reported a significant improvement in the degree of curvature when individuals practiced a pose called Vasisthasana (side plank) on the convex side of the curve every day for an average of 90 seconds. This initial study, although it had some methodological limitations, found an average 32 percent improvement overall and a nearly 41 percent improvement in compliant subjects and put yoga on the map in the medical world as a viable, non-invasive solution to scoliosis and the complications that can arise from this condition. Still, there is much to be seen, studied, and learned about the positive impact that yoga and, more specifically, yoga therapy, can have on patient outcomes in many areas including their physical limitations, pain scale, functional mobility, and quality of life.

Purna Yoga involves a great deal more than just physical postures, and it is important to understand this concept if you choose to take a yoga therapy approach towards evolving your spine. Yoga therapy is a means towards healing from all pain and suffering, not just in the physical realm, but in the psychological, emotional, and spiritual areas of your life as well. This is one of the reasons that it is so tricky to conduct a scientific research study on the benefits of yoga for scoliosis. From a yoga therapy perspective, each treatment plan must be individually tailored, and so the outcomes you may experience, especially emotionally and spiritually, are often not measurable by modern scientific standards.

# Anatomy of the curve

Before you can use Purna Yoga to help you with scoliosis, it is important to understand what it is and how it impacts your movement. Scoliosis is defined as an S-shaped curve, or sideways curve, that usually develops in growing children before puberty. Most often, the cause is unknown and the condition is called "idiopathic scoliosis." Scoliosis can be structural or functional and it is important to distinguish the two. Structural scoliosis refers to the actual shape of the curve due to changes in the skeletal structure and includes a sideways curve and rotation in the vertebrae. Functional scoliosis is a sideways curve that develops due to an imbalance in the pull of the muscles and is related mostly to activities that encourage an uneven pull on the spine or muscle spasm. Functional scoliosis does not include a rotational component in the spine; it is easier, therefore, to normalize, as treatment entails finding balance in the muscles and surrounding tissues in order to eliminate an uneven pull on the spine. With structural scoliosis, the anomaly is more challenging to treat as it stems not just from the muscles but from the spine itself.

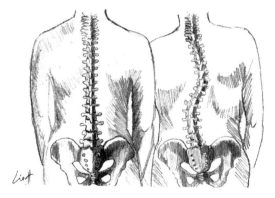

*Figure 1.1 Scoliosis*

A scoliotic curve can be found in the upper or lower back and consists of a primary curve and often a secondary, or compensatory curve as well. The body, in its infinite wisdom and desire to achieve balance at all costs, finds a way to make sure that the head remains centered. In order to do this, the spine—like a delicate strand of pearls—adapts by curving in the opposite direction of the primary curve. I find this a quite beautiful illustration of how the body is seeking balance at all times.

**a.**

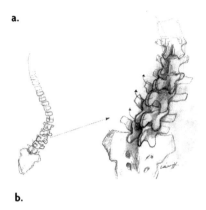

**b.**

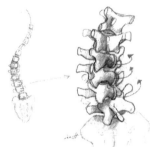

*Figure 1.2 a. Curve bent to the left with right rotational component b. Curve bent to the right with left rotational component*

The second and very important aspect of scoliosis to understand is the rotational component. While most individuals understand the sideways bend of the curve, fewer realize that when a curve bends to one side, the vertebrae are actually rotated to the opposite direction. That is to say that if the curve is bent to the left, the vertebrae will be rotated to the right. Conversely, if the curve is bent to the right, the individual segments of the spine (the vertebrae) will be rotated to the left (see Figure 1.2 a., b.).

The rotational component of the vertebrae is what gives rise to what we call a "rib hump" which is often visible on individuals when they move into a forward bend (see Figure 1.3).

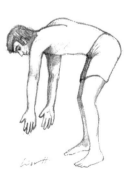
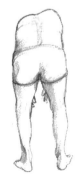

*Figure 1.3 Forward bend illustrating rib hump*

In medical terminology, the curve is named for the convex side, or the side where there is a hump. For example, if your curve is side bent to the left, the convex side will be on the right and so will the hump. Therefore, this is called a right scoliosis. Similarly, if your curve is side bent to the right, the convex side will be on the left and so will the hump due to the vertebral rotation to the left side.

The best place to begin a course of treatment is with a complete postural evaluation by a physiotherapist, orthopedic doctor, or osteopath, so that you will have the information you need to understand your curve. Here are some questions you may want to ask.

1. Where is your primary curve? *Thoracic, lumbar, or a double curve (equal curve in both the lumbar and thoracic area)*

2. Which type of curve is it? *Functional or structural*

3. On which side is the hump? *Right or left scoliosis*

When you know these three answers, you will have enough information to help guide you in your next steps. If you have a right scoliosis with right rotation of the vertebrae then twisting to the right in yoga will feel natural for you. However, when twisting to the left, you may find that there is an obvious blockage, or restriction. This is biomechanical and it is important to avoid allowing anyone to force or adjust you into a twist as it can cause compression that results in inflammation in the spine. When dealing with scoliosis, you have to *respect the curve* and work with its nuances in order to create length without any compression. In addition, if you take group yoga classes, it is probably best to tell your teacher about your scoliosis and any issues that may cause limitations and/or discomfort.

There are three main types of scoliosis, as noted in (1) above. Knowing which one of these three you have will help you move forward with your treatment as well. It is good to visualize the different curvatures so that you get a good understanding of what each type of curve looks like.

1. Thoracic curve—a C-curve that affects the upper back

2. Lumbar—a C-curve that affects the lower back

3. Double curve—e.g. left thoracic, right lumbar or right thoracic, left lumbar—a double major curve or S-curve that is equal in both the thoracic and lumbar spine

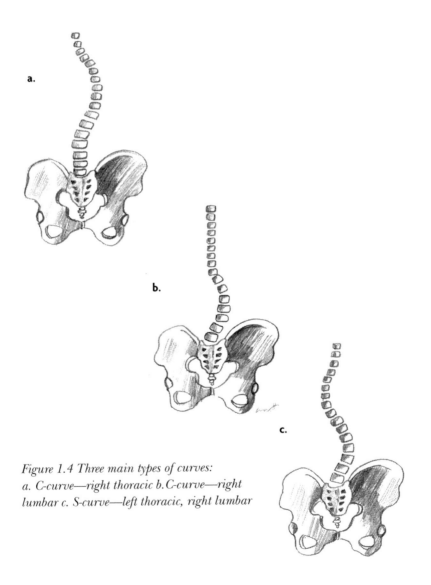

*Figure 1.4 Three main types of curves:*
*a. C-curve—right thoracic b. C-curve—right*
*lumbar c. S-curve—left thoracic, right lumbar*

Once you understand your curve and have a better understanding of what you are dealing with, you will need to establish your treatment protocol. In the coming chapters, we will define a ten-step approach that will help you re-align your body, decrease pain from compression due to the curvature, and prevent the curve from progressing further.

The treatment approach is as follows:

1. Release muscular tension

2. Open your hips

3. Find your mountain pose

4. Strengthen the convex side

5. Lengthen the concave side

6. Create length and symmetry

7. Traction your spine

8. Practice acceptance and surrender

9. Quiet your mind

Practicing all these elements, in this order, will help you establish a short daily practice that will be easy to incorporate into your life no matter how busy you are. The long-term results will not only improve your curve, but could also transform your life.

And there is one last rule that you should follow regularly:

10. *Rest when you need it!*

People with scoliosis tend to be pulled in many different directions and have a hard time listening to their own needs. If this rings true for you, take the time out to allow yourself to nourish your body and your soul. Notice if you are taking on too much and literally "carrying the weight of the world on your shoulders." Value your time off and prioritize the activities that most nourish and sustain you. This is the most important principle of all.

# CHAPTER 2

# Understanding Yoga Therapy

A common misunderstanding in the western approach to yoga is a tendency to emphasize the physical postures (asana) only. The physical postures are in fact just one aspect of a system that offers an eight-fold path towards transformation and liberation from suffering. If you decide to use Purna Yoga as a means towards healing, you will need to keep in mind your intention of using the physical practice as one aspect of the bigger picture. Just doing the asana can provide a nice system of stretching and strengthening, but this is not considered the practice of yoga in its wider context. While the physical poses will indeed relieve back pain and can help normalize your spinal curve, you will need to go deeper to experience the inner peace that you may be longing for. To understand the ancient wisdom of yoga as therapy it is important to understand the complete system, which includes the eight limbs of yoga. These are: the yamas and niyamas, asana, pranayama, pratyahara, dharana, dhyana, and samadhi.

The first two limbs of yoga, the yamas and niyamas, refer to the ethical practice of yoga and are the foundations upon which you are to begin a physical practice.

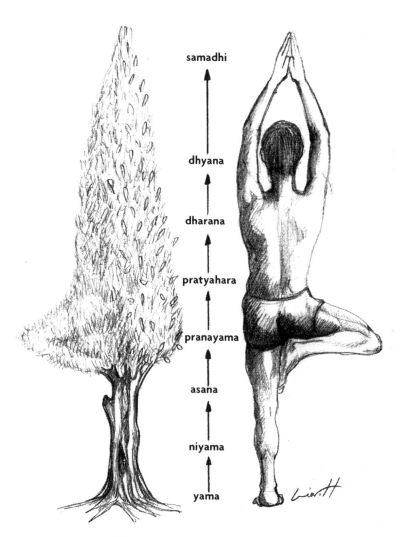

samadhi

dhyana

dharana

pratyahara

pranayama

asana

niyama

yama

*Figure 2.1 The eight limbs of yoga*

# 1. The yamas

## *Ahimsa—Non-violence*

Non-violence can be interpreted in many ways including your behavior towards others, the planet, and ultimately yourself. In the context of scoliosis, this is one of the most important precepts. Within it, I believe, lies the secret to working with this condition. Do you view your curve as something that you need to "fight" or "counter"? Do you view your body as "crooked" and in need of "straightening"? Are you willing to try a different approach that embodies more acceptance and kindness at every turn? If you view your curve as separate from you, then it is an entity that needs to be corrected and straightened out. It becomes something that you see as a "problem" or "damaged" and, therefore, you might approach the problem with a violent attitude, or an aggressive wish to "fix" it. While bracing and surgery can be beneficial to individuals with significant curves, it can sometimes be an all too violent approach that the body will ultimately reject. However, whether these treatments are needed or not, you can still choose another way to work with your body. You can work with the curve, and incorporate physical postures (asana), including breath, awareness, and a sense of softness in your practice. You can trust that, if you provide the right conditions, the spine will find its balance. You can find what works for you and know that you have the tools to help yourself without the need for external devices. You can choose kindness over aggression, peace instead of violence.

## *Satya—Truthfulness*

Being honest is essential in order to live with the integrity that is expected on the yogic path. The problem is that sometimes the hardest person to be honest with is you. You may want to check in and notice if you are respecting your body. Are you pushing too hard in your physical activity or are you disconnected from your body because you just don't want to deal with it? Do you really not have time to exercise or are you making excuses? Being honest also means knowing your limitations in postures and choosing the best variation in the pose for your body, regardless of what the rest of the class is doing. Being honest means making sure that a teacher is not pushing you too hard so that you do not hurt yourself. If you commit to regular movement with a qualified teacher, your curve will improve—there is no doubt about it. But the more truthful you are about your condition and your abilities, the better your progress will be.

## Asteya—Non-stealing

Stealing comes from the belief that "I do not have enough," that "I am not provided for" and that, therefore, I need to take from someone else in order to survive. In scoliosis, you may look at others and wish that your spine was straighter, or that you could accomplish a pose with as much ease as another who may have a different range of motion. Embodying asteya means being content with what you have and working within that framework. This can eliminate a great deal of unnecessary pain and suffering.

## Brahmacharya—Moderation or Non-excess

This yama refers to knowing how much of anything you need and letting go of the rest. It is about being moderate in everything, especially in expending your creative energy. It is about pausing and making choices about where to put your efforts from a higher place rather than following your lower instincts or base desires.

## Aparigraha—Non-possessiveness or Non-coveting

The root of this yama is the realization that you are not your body. You cannot be attached to looking like others or getting hung up on what seems perfect on the outside. We are not symmetrical beings, nor are we meant to be. Everyone has his or her own challenges, whether visible on the outside or not. Continue to approach others with compassion and loving kindness and you will attract that kind of acceptance into your life. Do not envy others and just do your work. You may find that your struggles are exactly what you need to move ahead with a purposeful life.

# 2. The niyamas

## Saucha—Purity—Cleanliness, Neatness

Yoga is very much about order. You strive to set up a practice space for yourself and keep it neat. You create and stick to a schedule. The idea is that if there is order in your physical space, there is order in your mind and your inner world. It is hard to remain grounded when your environment is chaotic and your mind scattered.

## Santosha—Contentment

This concept of being satisfied with what you are and have is quite different from what most of us call "happiness" today. It is about cultivating an attitude of acceptance, regardless of external circumstances. While there may be pain or discomfort, you can still choose contentment. My Purna Yoga teacher, Aadil Palkhivala, tells a story of his visit to a chiropractor after an acute bout of lower back pain. The pain was severe and Aadil went to the health practitioner to help him re-align his spine. The chiropractor asked him many questions all of which he answered in a pleasant tone with a gentle smile. Towards the end of the visit the doctor looked puzzled and spoke.

"May I ask you a question?"

"Certainly," replied my teacher.

"A lot of people visit my office who are experiencing a great deal of pain. I wonder how you can still smile when all this is going on?"

Aadil smiled again and answered softly, "I have no choice about the pain, but I do have the choice to be happy."

## Tapas—Self-discipline

Do your exercises! Nothing will change if you don't do them, just as you could not lose weight only by saying you want to instead of changing your diet and exercise regime. In order to experience the benefits, you need to commit to your program and stick with it. Give it six weeks at least to see your best results. Don't question it, get up each day and do your practice. Discipline is considered the fire needed to create transformation. Without the fire, you cannot turn metal into gold. "Yoga is 99 percent practice and 1 percent theory" was a favorite saying of the founder of Ashtanga yoga, Guru Pattabhi Jois.

## Svadhyaya—Self-study

Yoga asks you not only to practice, but to observe yourself during the practice. As you move through the program notice your reactions, judgments, and/or resistance that arise. Do you feel some hesitation about doing some of the exercises—or all? Are there certain ones you avoid and others that you become attached to? Notice where you feel tight in the poses, then breathe more into those areas. Notice where you hold your breath. Notice your posture. Does judgment come up? Self-hatred? What are the beliefs you hold about your body that arise when you start paying attention? Self-study is not about changing anything, but rather about observing and being with what is. You will not be able to change until you notice your patterns of thinking and response. These can be so ingrained in your subconscious that you have no idea what you are thinking and doing. When you stop and pay attention, things start to change.

## Ishvara Pranidhana—Surrender

This one is tough. Yoga asks us to do the practice and then not to be attached to results. You are invited to be happy with what is and to do the work without focusing on the outcome. Ultimately, major changes may occur when you begin the program, and then things might balance out, and you may experience a plateau. You may suffer a setback. Either way, you wake up, practice gratitude for all you have, for your body the way it is, and do the work. Let go of the results and surrender. While it may seem counterintuitive, this attitude will assure you of the peace that you seek.

# 3. Asana—The physical postures

Asana is the third limb of yoga and refers to the physical practice that can help you relieve physical pain and improve your ability to focus and be still. The aim of asana is to align the spine so that you can sit without pain for meditation. If the body hurts, you cannot focus on anything other than the pain. In order to progress past the physical body and move towards more meditation, yoga provides you with tools to improve your posture, keep your spine mobile, and improve your breathing capacity. As physicians at the Mayo Clinic note on their website (2015), one of the most common complications of scoliosis is a restriction of the rib cage, and this can lead to respiratory infections. Learning how to increase the expansion of your rib cage and, consequently, your lungs, will help improve oxygenation, and this, in turn, can help you to relieve tension in muscles surrounding the back and neck.

# 4. Pranayama—Mastery of the breath

The aim of asana (physical postures) is to prepare the body for pranayama, using the breath to tap into increased vitality or *life force.*

The last four stages of the eight-fold path refer to the stages of meditation:

# 5. Pratyahara—Withdrawal of the senses

Your mind leaves sensation behind.

# 6. Dharana—Single pointed focus

By fixing the mind on something, you create a state of concentration.

# 7. Dhyana—A deep state of meditation

This means perfect contemplation, and the experience of equanimity and awareness without attachment.

# 8. Samadhi—Oneness

This is the ultimate aim of yoga, achieving a spiritual state of pure consciousness or oneness with all that is.

When we talk about yoga as therapy, we are referring to all the tools that yoga can offer to end pain and suffering on multiple levels. Yoga therapy also works within the framework of the five koshas—translated as layers or sheaths—that incorporate all five aspects of being (see Figure 2.2). In yoga philosophy, the koshas refer to the physical body (*annamaya kosha*), the energy body (*pranamaya kosha*), the mental/emotional body (*manomaya kosha*), the wisdom body or intellectual body (*vijnanamaya kosha*), and the bliss body (*anandamaya kosha*).

The idea underlying the koshas is simple: everything is connected. You may already know this from your scoliosis, a condition that can make you aware that one vertebra affects the next and the next and then has a ripple effect, causing an impact on all parts of the body. Any block or limitation in one layer or kosha will affect the other, thereby creating disharmony in the individual.

To work on all five koshas, you will use physical postures, breath, intention, awareness, examination of your core beliefs, meditation, and visualization as part of the treatment plan. When used in unison and incorporated into daily life, *as a way of life*, then complete pain relief and well-being are at your fingertips.

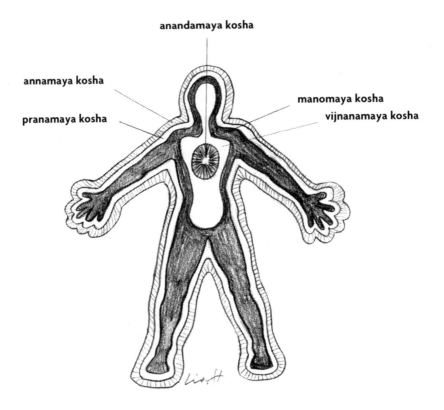

anandamaya kosha

annamaya kosha

pranamaya kosha

manomaya kosha

vijnanamaya kosha

*Figure 2.2 The five koshas*

This book is a first step. You will learn the basic principles for working with your scoliosis and some helpful exercises that have been shown to improve the curvature and release tension in the spine and surrounding muscles and joints. But I highly recommend that you go beyond these pages and seek out an experienced Purna Yoga teacher or yoga therapist who can work with you privately or in a group setting to take your practice further. With the understanding that the body is a gateway to the soul, you will experience far more than symptomatic relief of your scoliosis. You will find a new way to be in your body with joy, ease, and acceptance for the rest of your life.

# The Practice
## PART II

## CHAPTER 3

# Releasing Tension

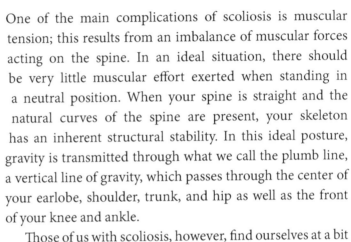

One of the main complications of scoliosis is muscular tension; this results from an imbalance of muscular forces acting on the spine. In an ideal situation, there should be very little muscular effort exerted when standing in a neutral position. When your spine is straight and the natural curves of the spine are present, your skeleton has an inherent structural stability. In this ideal posture, gravity is transmitted through what we call the plumb line, a vertical line of gravity, which passes through the center of your earlobe, shoulder, trunk, and hip as well as the front of your knee and ankle.

Those of us with scoliosis, however, find ourselves at a bit of a disadvantage because the S-shaped curve takes us out of the ideal plumb line. With this imbalance, other muscles that were not designed to be active all day long are asked to hold us up against gravity. The muscles of the concave side of the curve become shortened and tight and continue to exert a pull on the spine. The muscles on the convex side of the curve are stretched out and also, therefore, become weak. In order to keep ourselves upright at all costs, our bodies will recruit various other muscles to take over the task of standing.

*Figure 3.1 The plumb line—optimal postural alignment*

This often causes pain and tension in many areas of the spine. Tired muscles are being overworked or asked to do a job for which they were not originally designed.

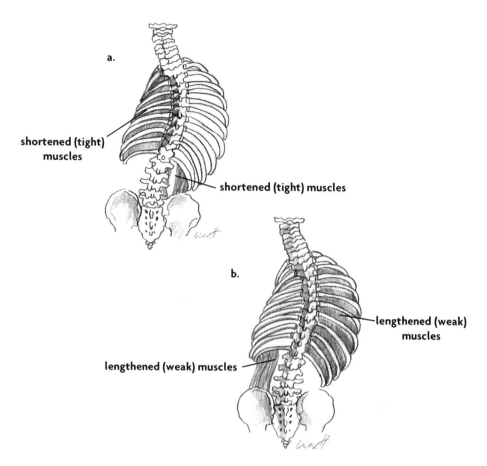

*Figure 3.2 Pull of muscles in scoliosis: a. on concave side b. on convex side*

In Purna Yoga, many techniques can be applied to help release tension in the muscles of the trunk, tension that often contributes to chronic pain. Before we can make changes to your spine, we need to release the pull of these muscles so that your spine can begin to straighten out. One of my favorite sequences to help release tension in the muscles and fascia that run from the base of the skull all the way down to the tailbone is the *Purna Yoga Morning Series*. Developed by Purna Yoga founder Aadil Palkhivala, this series consists of eight postures, all done while lying on the back.

The emphasis of the morning series is on increasing mobility and flexibility with shorter holds and movement that is coordinated with the breath. The eight postures are repeated a number of times on each side. The effort is exerted on the exhalation while your body is completely at rest during the inhalation. The beautiful thing about this sequence is that it can take less than five minutes to do, or you can turn it into a 20- to 30-minute practice depending on how much time you have.

# Release muscular tension
## *The Morning Series*

This warm-up can be used at the beginning of a practice, or in bed upon waking; it releases tension in the spine and increases mobility.

### 1. FULL BODY STRETCH

Lie on your back and take your arms overhead with the palms facing up towards the ceiling. Keep your legs together and straight. Take a deep inhalation as you relax in this position, filling your lungs with oxygen. While exhaling, reach through your fingertips and press out through your heels, flexing your toes towards your head. As you inhale, relax completely, allowing your whole body to let go. Exhaling, stretch through your heels and fingertips again and lift your lower belly towards your chin.

Lifting the lower belly entails drawing your belly button towards your spine and upward in order to engage the deeper abdominal muscles which, in turn, protect the lower back. Exhaling, do the full body stretch again, this time moving the buttocks and sitting bones towards the heels. This action will take the arch out of your lower back in order to lengthen your spinal muscles.

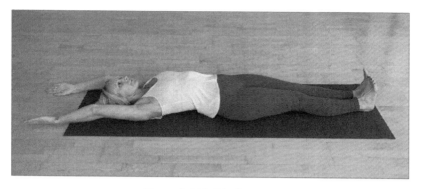

*Figure 3.3 Full body stretch*

## FULL BODY STRETCH: SUMMARY OF INSTRUCTIONS

- Lie on your back.

- Reach your arms overhead with palms facing upward (you can place a pillow under the arms if they do not reach the floor).

- Relax on the inhalation.

- Exhaling, reach your fingers overhead and press out through your heels with your toes flexed.

- Lift your lower belly towards your chin.

- Move your sitting bones towards your heels.

- Repeat three to nine times.

### 2. ANKLE PUMPS AND ANKLE CIRCLES

Keep your arms overhead or, alternatively, place the arms alongside your body. Take a deep breath in and, as you exhale, point your toes away from you and then reverse by flexing the toes back towards the face. Point and flex the toes as many times as possible while exhaling and relax as you take a deep breath in.

The aim of this exercise is to relax your upper back, neck, and entire spine as much as possible so that your whole body rocks as you pump the ankles. This requires an element of letting go. Notice where you tend to hold your tension and try to relax so that your whole body rocks with each ankle pump. Your neck and head should even be moving along with the movement of the ankles. Repeat three to nine times.

Next, make large circles with your ankles while keeping the feet together. Go through the full range of motion available to you, both feet circling in the same direction on the exhalation, while keeping the rest of your body relaxed. Do the ankle circles to the right and to the left, relaxing on the inhalation and moving on the exhalation. Repeat three to nine times.

## ANKLE PUMPS: SUMMARY OF INSTRUCTIONS

- Place your arms overhead or as an alternative, rest your arms alongside the torso.

- Take a deep breath in.

- While exhaling, point and flex the feet, allowing the whole body to rock with the movement.

- Relax on the inhalation.

- Repeat three to nine times.

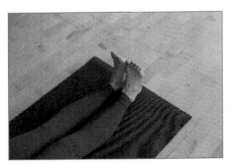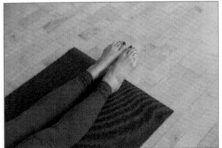

*Figure 3.4 a. Ankle pumps*

# ANKLE CIRCLES: SUMMARY OF INSTRUCTIONS

- Place your arms overhead or, as an alternative, rest your arms alongside the torso.

- Take a deep breath in.

- While exhaling, circle both ankles to the right with the feet together, allowing the whole body to rock with the movement.

- Relax on the inhalation.

- Exhaling, circle ankles to the left.

- Repeat three to nine times—alternating ankle circles to the right and left.

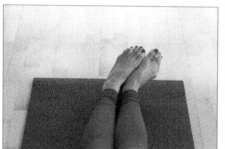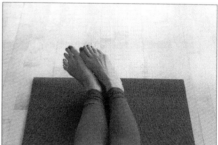

*Figure 3.4 b. Ankle circles*

### 3. STRAIGHT-LEG TWIST

Continue lying on your back. Stretch your right arm out to the side, at shoulder height, with your palm facing upward. Place your left hand on top of your right shoulder. With straight legs, lift your right leg and place your right Achilles tendon in the webbing between the first and second toe of your left foot. Exhaling, lift the lower belly towards your chin as you twist your pelvis to the left, bringing the toe of your right foot towards the floor on your left side. Press through both heels to keep the spine long. At the same time, rotate your head to the right and push your right shoulder down with your left hand. Inhaling, come back to neutral and switch legs. Repeat on the other side while exhaling.

It is important to keep the legs straight for this variation, which requires activation of both legs, so keep both knees straight during the twist and press out strongly through the heels. This will protect your lower back. Don't worry about how far you can twist. Just do your best with the legs straight. Keep your shoulders on the ground as you twist at all times. Keep lifting your lower belly as you press out through the heels to increase length in the lumbar spine. Only look over the opposite shoulder in this twist if it does not bother your neck. If there is neck pain and/or tension, keep your chin in line with your chest throughout the twist.

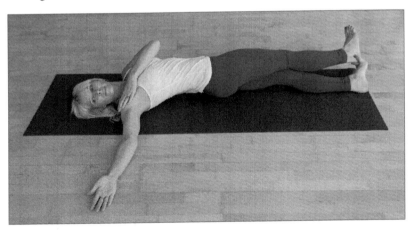

*Figure 3.5 Straight-leg twist*

## STRAIGHT-LEG TWIST:
## SUMMARY OF INSTRUCTIONS

- Extend your right arm out at shoulder height and place left hand on your right shoulder.

- Place your right heel in between the first and second toe of your left foot.

- Inhale.

- As you exhale, twist to the left, keeping the right shoulder on the ground.

- Press out through your heels and lift your lower belly.

- Inhaling, come back onto your back and rest.

- Switch your arms and legs and repeat by twisting to the right on the next exhalation.

- Repeat three to nine times alternating between the right and left sides.

## 4. BENT-LEG TWIST

Bend your right knee and place your foot on the outside of your left knee. Then place your left hand on the outside of your right knee and bring your knee towards the ground. Try to get the knee as close to the ground as possible, allowing your right shoulder to come off the floor. Straighten your right arm and reach out through your fingertips with the palms up, keeping your arm at shoulder level.

Take a deep breath in and as you exhale push out through the bottom heel, lift the lower belly and twist the upper body back to the right.

Keeping the bottom leg straight and active is important in order to protect your lower back in this pose. The twist should come more from your upper back area as you try to reach your shoulder towards the ground. If there is any back pain, just allow your right knee to come off the floor until there is no more discomfort. Keep your lower belly lifted to protect your lower back as well.

If you are fairly flexible, you can gaze over the right shoulder but if there is any neck discomfort, keep the head in line with the center of your chest.

Repeat three to nine times each side, alternating from right to left.

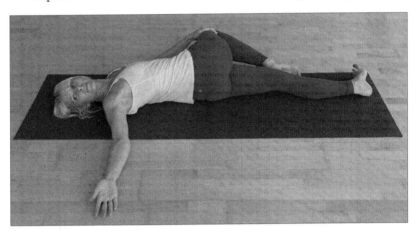

*Figure 3.6 Bent-leg twist*

## BENT-LEG TWIST: SUMMARY OF INSTRUCTIONS

- Bend your right knee and place your foot on the outside of your left leg.

- Hold the outside of your knee with the opposite hand and bring your knee to the ground.

- Push out through your bottom heel and lift your lower belly.

- Stretch through your right fingertips to open the front of your chest.

- Rotate your rib cage to the right, increasing mobility in your thoracic spine.

## 5. SINGLE KNEE TO CHIN

Start lying on your back with your legs straight. Exhaling, bend your right knee and pull it into your chest. Clasp your leg just below the knee on the shin. Keeping your belly soft, pull the leg into your chest as you bring your chin towards your knee. You may coax the bent leg towards the right armpit if there is pain in the hip. As you inhale, release the leg as you bring your head to the floor. Repeat on the left side and alternate for three to nine repetitions.

The intention of this posture is to lengthen and soften the back muscles, not to strengthen the core, so focus on lengthening the back of the body rather than contracting the abdominals. If there is any pain in the neck, keep the head on the ground during this exercise.

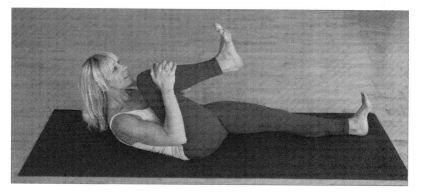

*Figure 3.7 Single knee to chin*

### SINGLE KNEE TO CHIN: SUMMARY OF INSTRUCTIONS

- Inhale deeply.

- Exhaling, bring your knee to your chest.

- Lift your head (if there is no neck pain) and bring your chin to your knee.

- Release and repeat on the left side.

- Repeat for three to nine cycles.

## 6. DOUBLE KNEE TO CHIN

Start with either straight legs or with your knees bent and feet on the floor. If you have back pain, I recommend that you keep your knees bent throughout the exercise. Exhaling, bring both knees into your chest, wrapping your arms around your legs and interlacing your fingers to guide the legs towards the chest. Bring your chin up towards your knees. Inhaling, release.

As in the last posture, the emphasis here is on stretching the muscles of the back and neck, not on contracting the abdominals.

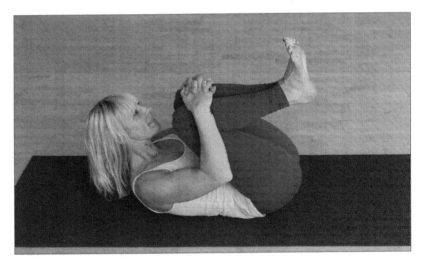

*Figure 3.8 Double knee to chin*

---

### DOUBLE KNEE TO CHIN: SUMMARY OF INSTRUCTIONS

- Start with straight legs or bent knees (for those with back pain).

- Exhaling, hug both knees in towards the chest.

- Lift the chin up towards the knees.

- Release on the inhalation.

- Repeat three to nine times.

## 7. SIDE ROLLS

Pull your knees into your chest, wrapping your arms around your legs and holding onto your forearms. Keep your head on the floor and in line with the center of your chest throughout the exercise. Exhaling, roll to the right side, going only as far as you can without reaching the floor, and then roll back up. Inhaling, rest in the center and then roll to the left side and back up while exhaling. Repeat three to nine times on each side.

As you roll to each side, feel the muscles that run along your spine being massaged by the floor as if cookie dough were being smoothed out by a rolling pin. Control the movement by using your abdominals to prevent yourself from dropping the knees to the floor at any point. This pose helps to release tight muscles along the spine. If you notice an area that is tighter or slightly painful, take your time rolling over that area and work into the tightness.

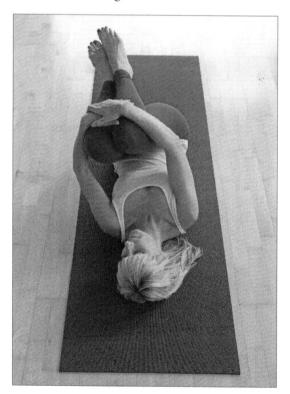

*Figure 3.9 Side rolls*

## SIDE ROLLS: SUMMARY
## OF INSTRUCTIONS

- Lie on your back and bring both knees into your chest, holding onto your forearms or wrists.

- Keep your head in line with your chest and inhale while lying on your back.

- Exhaling, slowly roll to the right, controlling the movement without touching the ground; return back to neutral.

- On the next exhalation, roll to the left and back up to neutral.

Repeat three to nine times on each side, alternating from right to left, massaging your back muscles on the ground throughout the movement.

## 8. HAMSTRING STRETCH

Place a yoga strap just above the heel of your right foot and bring your leg up, keeping the knee extended. Straighten your left leg as much as possible, as you flex your toes and press your left heel away from your head. Keep your head and shoulders on the floor. Contract your right thigh muscle and straighten your right knee. If you cannot straighten the right leg, release the leg until the point where you can extend your knee. The height of the leg is less important than the extension of the knee so don't worry about reaching a 90-degree angle. As long as you feel a nice stretch behind your right thigh, you are doing it correctly. Hold here for three breaths and then repeat on the left side. Do three to nine rounds, alternating legs.

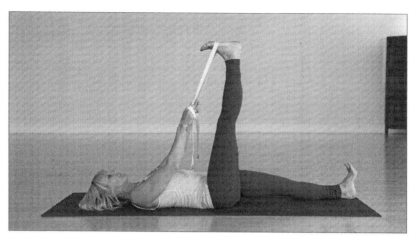

*Figure 3.10 Hamstring stretch*

## HAMSTRING STRETCH: SUMMARY OF INSTRUCTIONS

- Place a strap above the heel of your right foot and lift your leg.

- Straighten your left leg and push out through your left heel.

- Contract your right thigh muscle and straighten your right knee, feeling a nice stretch in your hamstrings, on the rear side of the right thigh.

- Keep your frontal hip bones (the bony prominences on the anterior pelvis) at the same level.

- Hold for three breaths and repeat with the left leg.

- Repeat three to nine times, alternating right and left legs.

## 9. RETURN TO FULL BODY STRETCH

To complete the series, finish with the same pose you started with—the full body stretch. Repeat three to nine times stretching the whole body while exhaling.

## Open Your hips

After the morning series, I recommend that you practice one very important posture designed to open your hips. This hip opener will directly affect your ability to stand up straighter with less compression in the spine. It is a subtle pose, but very effective if you struggle with back pain. The posture is hip internal rotation and it is one of the only postures that move the hip into full internal rotation. In addition to increasing your range of motion in the hip joint, this pose lengthens and releases the iliopsoas muscle, a powerful hip flexor attaching directly to the front of the lumbar spine and discs. Releasing tension in this muscle allows your spine to lengthen naturally creating a sense of lightness and ease with standing.

In general, hip openers are essential for overall back health and there are many options found in a regular yoga practice. Begin with this hip opener, but don't stop here. You will want to open the hips in all possible ranges of motion as most muscles around the hips connect to the pelvis and sacrum directly affecting the alignment of your spine.

For best results, I highly recommend practicing the full "Purna Yoga Hip Opening Series" which is outlined in my first book, *Yoga for a Happy Back: A Teacher's Guide to Spinal Health through Yoga Therapy.*

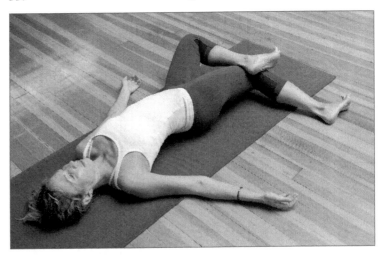

*Figure 3.11 Hip internal rotation*

## HIP INTERNAL ROTATION
## (DURYODHANĀSANA)

Increases internal rotation in the hip joint and stretches the Iliopsoas muscle.

- Lie on your back with your feet on the floor and knees bent at a 90-degree angle.

- Step your right foot over to the right one shin length. Flex both feet, and then bring your right knee down towards your left ankle. Next, lift your left foot and place your left ankle on the outside of your right thigh just above your knee.

- Let your right buttock come off the ground in this pose but make sure to lift your lower belly in order to maintain the integrity of the lumbar spine.

- *Important! If there is any pain in the right knee, place a block or blanket underneath your inner knee for support.*

- If there is no pain in your right knee joint, begin to move the knee away from the head so you focus on creating traction in the hip while in internal rotation. Do not press the knee towards the floor, emphasize length instead, but do let it drop downward on its own.

- Lengthen your thighbone away from your head as you pull your lower belly towards your head.

- Hold for nine breaths, and then switch sides.

Finally, coming off the ground, you have released tension in your back muscles and your hips; now you can practice standing in mountain pose (Tadasana).

## *Find your mountain pose*
### HOW TO STAND

The goal of Tadasana is to maintain the normal curves of the spine so the muscles that have been working hard to "hold you up against gravity" can relax as you find the optimal position where gravity can be absorbed by the skeleton and the muscles designed for postural control can be accessed and strengthened.

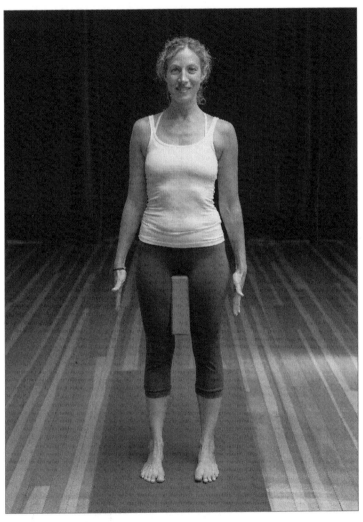

*Figure 3.12 Mountain pose (Tadasana)*

The key is to maintain a lower lumbar curve while keeping the back of the body long so that there is more space between each vertebra. This is called "axial extension" and occurs when you apply the following instructions:

- Place a block between your upper thighs and stand with your feet hip-width distance apart.

- Press all four corners of your feet into the earth, lifting your arches. This proper contact with the ground energizes the leg muscles and prevents pronation (flat feet) and supination (outwardly arched feet) so that the hips and knees are in proper alignment. In addition, the more you ground into the earth, the more you will lengthen, so think about *rooting down* in order to *lift*.

- Engage your quadriceps by lifting your kneecaps up into your thighs. It is essential to fire the quadriceps in standing so that your legs hold the weight of the body, not the lower back, which is the more vulnerable part.

- Squeeze the block with your inner thighs and lightly rotate your thighbones inward as if trying to push the block out the back. Relax the buttocks. Make sure that your knees point straight ahead even though your thighs are rolling inward.

- Maintaining the internal rotation of the thighs, locate your lower belly (the area between the navel and the pubic bone) and lift the lower belly towards your head. This action is very important for maintaining length in the lower back as well as stabilizing the core. As you lift the lower belly, you can feel the sacrum descending towards the earth. *DO NOT TUCK the tailbone.* Tucking only increases tension in the lower back and sacroiliac (SI joint) and causes a decreased lumbar curve.

- Move your shoulder blades away from your ears and lift your sternum. When you descend the shoulder blades, you help to open your chest and relax the upper trapezius (neck) muscle.

- Lengthen through the crown of your head. This creates length through the entire spine from the inside out and prevents forward head posture.

- Hold this properly aligned stance for one to two minutes. Release and repeat twice every hour.

## HOW TO SIT

Sitting can sometimes be the most painful position for students or clients with scoliosis, as it increases pressure on the lower back. You may find it hard to sit for an extended period of time or you may have a difficult time sitting on airplanes for long flights. Use this technique to sit with less compression in your spine and to build up your postural muscles.

- First, make sure your hips are above the knees (best at a 30-degree angle) and feet are planted on the floor.

- Roll up a towel or sheet and place the roll behind the sacrum. Please note that the roll should *not* be placed in the curve of your lumbar spine but at the very *base of the spine* behind the sacrum. This will help push your sacrum forward, allowing your lower back to maintain its natural lordotic curve.

- Place a belt or yoga strap around the center of your thighs so that the thighs are hip distance apart. This will help prevent your thighs from rolling out to the side, which can create more compression in the spine and compromise your natural lumbar curve.

- Sit in this position for a maximum of 30 to 60 minutes and then remove the strap, stand up, and walk around.

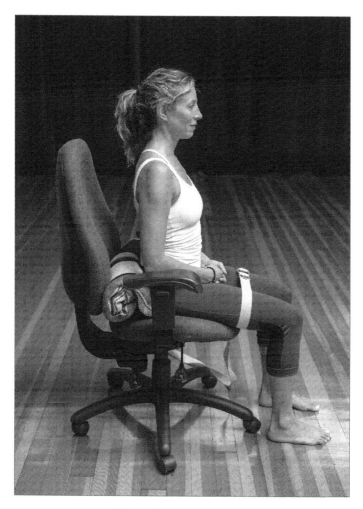

*Figure 3.13 Sitting posture*

When your muscles around the spine have released, you have begun
to experience the art of letting go. Perhaps you are also practicing with
a self-observing and non-judgmental attitude and are feeling more
hopeful and less attached to the results of your morning practice.
While this physical, mental, and emotional softening continues, you
are ready to move on to learning scoliosis-specific exercises that will
help you evolve your curvature and perhaps even normalize it.

# CHAPTER 4

# Elongation and Symmetry

Once you have released overall tension in the spine, the next step is to work on normalizing the curvature. To accomplish this, you will need the information gathered in Chapter 2 as to which type of curve you have and the direction of the curvature. Your goal here will be threefold:

1.  To strengthen the lengthened, weaker side of your curve.

2.  To lengthen the shortened, tighter side of your curve.

3.  To focus on general symmetry and optimal spinal alignment throughout the length of your spine.

## 1. Strengthening the weaker (convex) side

The pioneering study by Dr. Loren Fishman (2014) mentioned in Chapter 1 showed that practicing a single yoga pose for an average of one and a half minutes, five to seven days per week, improved the scoliotic curve by 32 percent. The progress in fully adherent patients—19 of 25 of those studied—was even more impressive. Their improvements of the curve, measured by the Cobb angle, increased to nearly 41 percent. For those with complex curves, meaning two opposing curves, the secondary curve also improved by 26 percent. While there is need for more high level research in the area of yoga and scoliosis, this study brings yoga to light as a potentially viable, non-invasive, non-traumatic, and low-cost option for individuals looking for alternatives. An improvement of this magnitude—32 percent on average—suggests that bracing and surgery can be avoided in some patients with scoliosis. This is really good news.

Let's review the anatomy described in Chapter 1, so that you can better identify your type of curvature. Remember that in scoliosis there is usually a primary and a secondary curve. If the primary curve is side bent to one side it will also be rotated to the opposite side. For example, if a primary lumbar curve is side bent to the right, it will be rotated to the left, and the secondary curve will be side bent to the left and rotated to the right (see Figure 1.2 a., b.). Also, we name the curve by the side of the convexity, so a curve that is side bent to the left is called a right scoliosis and vice versa.

Now you can identify which of the three main curves discussed in Chapter 1 describes yours: (1) thoracic; (2) lumbar; (3) complex or double curve, either right thoracic, left lumbar or left thoracic, right lumbar (see Figure 1.4). You may also need to consult with a physiotherapist or physician to understand the shape of your scoliosis.

At this point you should write down the type of curve you have, labeling it by the convex side. If you have a complex curve, list both. *For example: right thoracic C-curve, or complex right thoracic, left lumbar curve.*

Next, you will begin to practice the pose that proved so effective in normalizing scoliotic curves in Doctor Fishman's study, side plank pose (Vasisthasana). This posture can be practiced with variations, depending on what your needs are. You will be practicing asymmetrically, meaning only on one side, the convex side, so that you can balance out the scoliosis. *Because scoliosis is an asymmetrical condition, the only way to treat it is asymmetrically.* Follow the list below for the correct positioning of side plank pose.

If you have a lumbar or thoracic C-curve, practice traditional side plank as illustrated below (Figures 4.1, 4.2). If you have a double or complex curve, practice side plank with the leg lifted as illustrated in Figure 4.3.

## ━━━ REFERENCE LIST FOR SIDE PLANK ━━━

For a right lumbar scoliosis: right side

For a left lumbar scoliosis: left side

For a right thoracic scoliosis: right side

For a left thoracic scoliosis: left side

For complex curve—right lumbar curve, left thoracic curve: right side holding onto the left leg with the fingers or a strap

For complex curve—left lumbar curve, right thoracic curve: left side holding onto the right leg

---

## Side plank pose (Vasisthasana)

*Note:* Before practicing on your own I recommend that you work with a qualified yoga therapist to make sure that you are contracting the correct muscles during the exercise.

- Lie on the side that is indicated for you, with your back against a wall for support and your legs and feet stacked one on top of the other.

- Press your hand into the ground and extend your arm, lifting the trunk off of the floor. *Note:* Your arm should be at a 90-degree angle to the torso in the final variation of the posture.

- Lift your hips away from the floor so that your spine and pelvis are in one line.

- Lift your rib cage vertically towards the sky, shortening the bottom side of the torso. *Here we are looking to contract a muscle called the quadratus lumborum (QL) on the convex side of the curve. This muscle, when strengthened, will pull the spine away from the concavity towards a more neutral position (see Figure 4.1 a., b.).*

- Hold for as long as possible, building up to one and a half minutes or more.

- Repeat daily; results are best measured after a six-month period.

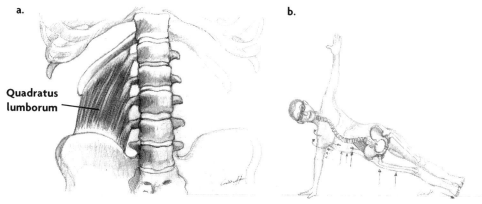

a.

**Quadratus lumborum**

b.

*Figure 4.1 a. Quadratus lumborum muscle (QL)*
*b. QL in side plank (illustration)*

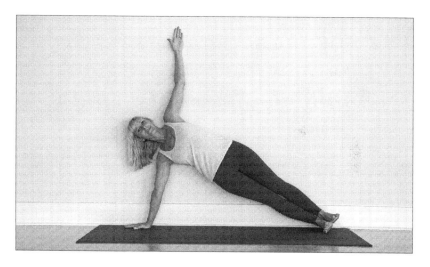

*Figure 4.1 c. Side plank (photo)*

This pose does require quite a bit of strength and balance, especially in the shoulder and wrist of the supporting hand. If the side plank is inaccessible to you due to limitations or injuries, here is a list of alternative options for you. Practice whichever one is best for you.

1.   Side plank on forearm is best done when there is pain in the wrist or conditions that are aggravated by bearing weight on an

extended arm, such as carpal tunnel syndrome or tennis elbow. If you have a shoulder injury it may feel more comfortable to practice with the forearm supported as well.

2.  Pressing into blocks with the upper arm takes some of the weight off of your bottom arm and unweights your shoulder joint even more.

3.  If it is still difficult to lift your pelvis off of the floor, let the legs rest on the ground and work on increasing strength by lifting your pelvis away from the floor in this position.

4.  Keeping your pelvis on the floor, lift the rib cage away from the ground. This will help you build strength on the lower side of the trunk.

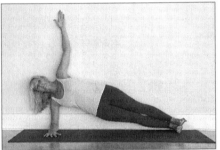 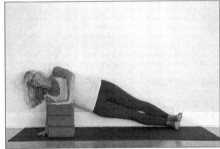

*Figure 4.2 Side plank: a. on forearm b. with top arm supported on blocks*

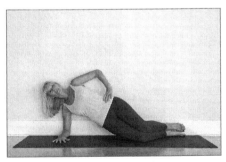 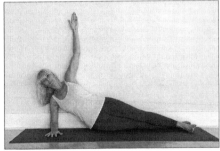

*Figure 4.2 c. With legs on the floor and knees bent*
*d. with legs and hips supported on the ground*

Finally, if you have a complex or double curve, you should practice side plank holding the top leg up with your free hand. Use your fingers to hold onto the big toe (for flexible folks) or use a strap to reach your foot. In both cases, focus on pulling with your top arm and side bending your upper trunk towards the sky as you pull the leg. Draw your top upper arm bone into the shoulder joint to maintain stability in the joint while holding onto your top leg. Straighten your knee by pressing the thighbone away from your head. Keep your top leg as straight as possible and in line with the rest of your body. Hold for as long as possible, working your way up to one and a half minutes.

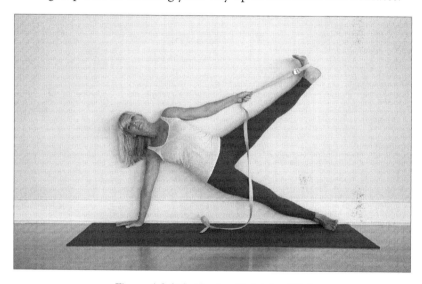

*Figure 4.3 Side plank with top leg lifted*

While side plank is more effective for scoliosis in the lumbar curve, a second pose can be used to target a thoracic curvature. This pose is half-moon pose (Ardha chandrasana) and is practiced more often with the convex side of your thoracic curve facing down. You want to work asymmetrically so that you normalize your scoliosis without putting too much pressure on one hip joint. Therefore, it is best to practice this posture on both sides but to hold longer and repeat twice as often with the convex side of your curve facing the ground. Refer to the box for the proper side to focus on.

**REFERENCE LIST FOR
HALF-MOON POSE**

For a right lumbar scoliosis: left side (left leg on the ground)

For a left lumbar scoliosis: right side

For a right thoracic scoliosis: right side

For a left thoracic scoliosis: left side

For complex curve—right lumbar curve, left thoracic curve: left side

For complex curve—left lumbar curve, right thoracic curve: right side

## Half-moon pose (Ardha chandrasana)

*Note:* Before practicing on your own I recommend that you work with a qualified yoga therapist to make sure that you are contracting the correct muscles during the exercise.

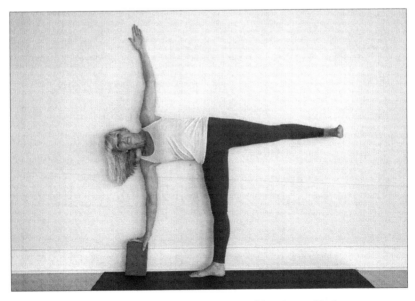

*Figure 4.4 Half-moon pose: a. pushing into a block*

## VARIATION 1—WITH A BLOCK
## (INSTRUCTED ON THE RIGHT SIDE)

- Begin standing against a wall and take your feet three and a half to four and a half feet wide.

- Turn your right toes out to 90 degrees and back toes in about 15 degrees, keeping the heel of the front leg in line with the center of the arch of your back foot.

- Place your hand on a block on the floor in front of your right foot and bend your right knee as you step your left foot in a bit.

- Shift the weight to your right leg and straighten your right knee as you lift your left leg off the ground. Use the wall for balance as needed.

- Press out through the left toe mounds and engage your quadriceps in both legs.

- Next, press strongly into the block with your right hand, contracting your lower torso muscles (the ones facing the floor) and lengthening your upper torso (the side of the rib cage that faces the ceiling).

- You must press your hand firmly into the block in a downward direction in order to activate the correct set of muscles. In this case, you want to activate the muscles that shorten your right rib cage in order to correct your thoracic curvature.

- Hold for one and a half to two minutes, then release.

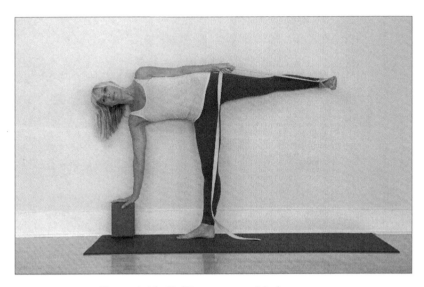

*Figure 4.4 b. Pulling a strap with the top arm*

### VARIATION 2—WITH A STRAP

- Move into half-moon pose as above and place a strap around your top foot.

- Instead of pushing down into the block, pull the strap with your top arm.

- The goal is to shorten or contract your lower torso muscles and to lengthen the upper side of your trunk as you pull the strap.

- Hold for one to one and a half minutes, then release.

# 2. Lengthening the tighter (concave) side

The next step to improving the curvature is to work on lengthening the side that is tight, which is the concave side of the curve. In addition to lengthening this side, you will want to add a little twist in order to balance out the rotational component of your scoliosis. I recommend that you practice the poses on both sides, but also that you do the side that is shortened twice as much. So, start and end with the limited or shortened side.

## —— REFERENCE LIST FOR STRETCHING ——

If you have a right scoliosis (lumbar or thoracic), you will stretch the left side of the trunk and twist to the left.

If you have a left scoliosis (lumbar or thoracic), you will stretch the right side of the trunk and twist to the right.

If you have a complex curve, you will do the poses equally on both sides.

## *Extended forward fold to one side*

- Begin on your hands and knees with your feet together and knees spread wide.

- Sit back on your heels as you walk your hands out in front, extending your elbows.

- Keep your wrists and elbows off of the floor, energizing your arms.

- Relax your neck muscles (upper trapezius) away from your ears. You should feel most of the work in your upper back muscles, not the neck.

- Now walk your hands to the side. The reference chart in the box will help you know which side you need to stretch—for example, for a right thoracic scoliosis, walk the hands to the right so that you stretch the left side of the torso.

- Next, add a slight twist to the opposite side. So, if you walk your hands to the right to stretch the left side of your trunk, twist your rib cage to the left.

- You may feel a stretch under the armpit or anywhere along the left side of your torso.

- Breathe into your rib cage on the side you are stretching, allowing the ribs to expand with each inhalation.

- Hold for a minimum of 30 seconds and repeat twice as much on the shortened side.

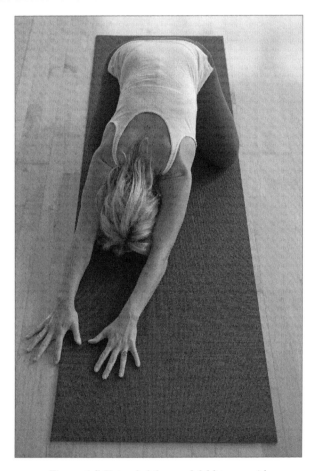

*Figure 4.5 Extended forward fold to one side*

## *Triangle pose (Trikonasana)*

There are many ways to practice this posture, as it is a foundational standing pose with many benefits for spine health. In this variation, you will focus on lengthening the shortened side (concave side) by practicing with different emphases on the two sides of the pose.

If your curve is convex to the right, the focus will be on lengthening the bottom side of the waist by placing a block or chair a few inches in front of your left leg. With scoliosis, the convex part of the curve will be facing the sky and the ribs stick out creating a rib hump. Your focus will be to lengthen the bottom side of your waist (the concave side of the curve) and to absorb your upper ribs (the convex side of the curve) into the body simultaneously (see Figure 4.6 a.).

For the same right convex curve, you will then practice on the second side by placing the block behind your right ankle and emphasize lengthening of the top of the trunk. In order to encourage even more opening of the concave side, stretch your top arm alongside your ear as you root your back heel into the ground (see Figure 4.6 b.). If your curve is convex to the left side, reverse the instructions below. If you have a double curve, work on correcting the primary (more prominent) curve.

**a.**                                         **b.**

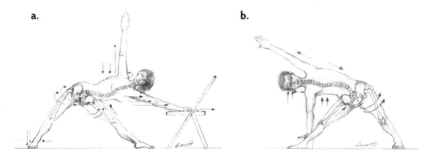

*Figure 4.6 a. Lengthening the bottom of the waist and absorbing the ribs into the body in triangle pose (for right scoliosis) with left leg forward b. Lengthening the top side of the waist in triangle pose (for right scoliosis) with right leg forward*

## TRIANGLE POSE (TRIKONASANA) INSTRUCTIONS
## (FOR RIGHT CONVEX CURVE)

- Step your legs approximately three and a half to four and a half feet apart.

- Turn your left foot out 90 degrees and turn your back toes in 15 degrees. Make sure that the heel of your front foot is in line with the center of the arch of your back foot.

- Engage your thigh muscles and lift your kneecaps, so that your legs are strong and supporting the spine.

- Reach out with the left hand so that you lengthen your spine. Place your hand on a chair or block in front of your left foot so that you lengthen the bottom side of the waist.

- Next, move your left ear away from your pelvis and absorb your upper ribs into your body as illustrated in Figure 4.6 a.

- Lift the right arm up in the air keeping the arm in line with your shoulder and in the same plane as the trunk.

- Rotate your rib cage towards the right and lift your lower belly up towards your chin.

- Hold for five to ten deep breaths.

- On the second side, take the same pose but place the block or chair slightly behind the right ankle. Here you will focus on lengthening the upper side of your waist.

- Reach overhead with your left arm alongside your left ear stretching through the fingertips to increase the length on your left side of the trunk as well.

- Root firmly into your back outer heel for support.

- Rotate the ribcage to the left as you lift your lower belly.

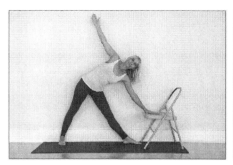 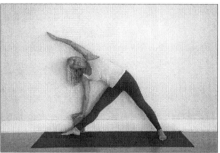

*Figure 4.7 Triangle pose (Trikonasana) for right convex curve: a. left leg forward (convex side up) b. right leg forward (convex side down)*

## *Extended side angle pose (Parsvakonasana)*

If you have a right scoliosis, thoracic or lumbar, practice twice as often on the shortened or concave side (left side) of the curve. If you have a complex or double curvature, practice equally on both sides.

- Step your legs out so that they are approximately four and a half to five and a half feet wide. The goal is that when you bend your front leg to a 90-degree angle, the knee should be directly above the ankle joint for stability (see Figure 4.8).

- Turn your right toes out to 90 degrees and your left toes in about five degrees. *For this variation you will be perpendicular to a wall with your right leg forward.*

- Make sure the heel of your front leg is in line with the center of the arch of your back foot.

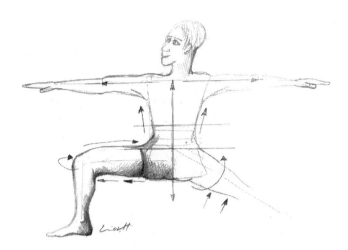

*Figure 4.8 Knee angle for front leg in extended side angle pose*

- Place your right forearm on the top of your right thigh, gently rotating your right thighbone backwards to keep the knee in line with the hip joint.

- Reach overhead with your left arm, palm facing down and allow your fingertips to reach the wall.

- Walk your fingers up the wall to increase length on the left side of your body, keeping your left ear close to your left upper arm bone.

- Root down firmly through your back outer heel.

- As you press through your back heel, stretch through the fingertips.

- Rotate your rib cage and torso to the left.

- Lift your lower belly towards your chin.

- Hold for five to ten breaths.

- Repeat twice as often on shortened side.

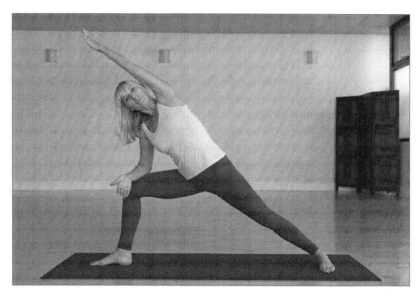

*Figure 4.9 Extended side angle pose (Parsvakonasana) for right convex curve*

## *Side-lying over bolster with rotation*

In this position, it is important to understand where the convexity of the curve is. You will place the bolster under the apex of your primary scoliotic curve for best results.

- For a right thoracic scoliosis, lie on your right side with the bolster or blanket roll under the right rib cage.

- Scissor the legs by taking your left leg forward and right leg back and press out through both heels, straightening out both knees.

- Exhaling, rotate the rib cage to the left.

- Reach out through the left fingertips keeping your elbow straight with your arm about 45 degrees above shoulder height.

- Hold for 30 seconds to one minute as tolerated.

- With every exhalation, focus on increasing left rotation of the thoracic spine and bringing your left shoulder closer to the ground.

- Make sure to press out through both heels as you lift your lower belly throughout this pose. This will help to stabilize your lower back.

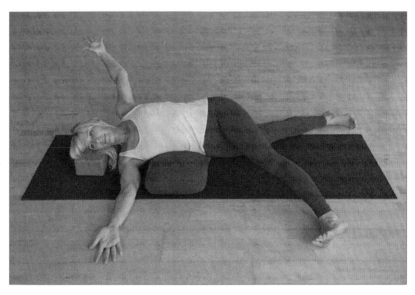

*Figure 4.10 Side-lying over bolster with trunk rotation*

# 3. Creating length and symmetry

The final and probably most important aspect of your physical practice will be to work on creating balance by elongating both sides of the trunk simultaneously. You want to teach your spine how to fire the muscles necessary to maintain proper alignment and posture. It is not enough simply to bend to the opposite side, but over the long term you want to encourage exercises that build up your general postural muscles and prevent the curve from getting worse. As gravity is always acting against you, you will need to commit to these postures regularly for maintenance and prevention. I have chosen a few simple postures that use a wall to help you accomplish this goal. I find that, if I am sitting for a long period of time, I like to get up and do these stretches during a break at a nearby wall. I even tend to do the first two in the back of the airplane when I travel long distances. You will be surprised at how easy it is to integrate a few minutes into your life during which you pamper your spine.

## *Half-forward bend (Ardha uttanasana)*

- Stand facing the wall and place your hands approximately waist height against the wall.

- Walk back slowly so that your arms are straight as you press into the wall with your palms.

- Make sure your feet are hip-width apart and your toes are pointing straight ahead.

- Contract the quadriceps strongly, lifting your kneecaps up as you press the tops of your thighs back.

- Move your pelvis away from your rib cage as you press into the wall with your hands, extending your elbows thereby creating traction in your lower back.

- Focus on lengthening the sides of the waist equally from your armpit to the top of your pelvis.

- If you have a rib hump, for example a right hump as in right thoracic scoliosis, then rotate your rib cage slightly to the left, absorbing the back ribs into the body. *It is helpful to have a yoga therapist or yoga instructor present to help guide you towards a more level spine.*

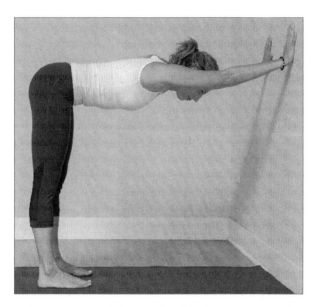

*Figure 4.11 Half-forward bend (Ardha uttanasana)*

## Half-pyramid pose (Ardha parsvottanasana)

- Start as above in a half-forward bend.

- Step your right leg forward about a foot and a half and step your left leg backward two feet.

- Turn your back foot out 45 degrees and press your heel into the ground.

- Square your hips by bringing the right outer hip back and moving your left hip forward.

- Lift the quadriceps in both legs and press the toe mounds firmly into the ground.

- Bring your inner thighs together.

- Focus on lengthening both sides of your waist equally and moving your pelvis away from the lower ribs.

- Absorb any rib hump into the body by rotating the rib cage to the opposite side of the hump.

- Lift your lower belly to protect your lower back.

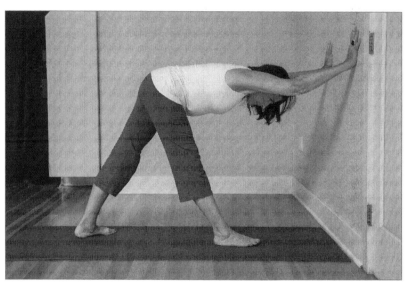

*Figure 4.12 Half-pyramid pose (Ardha parsvottanasana)*

## *Gate pose (Parighasana)*

- Come into a kneeling position with your left hip and thigh pressing against a wall.

- Extend your right leg out to the side and place the sole of your foot on the floor. The foot can be in line with your knee or turned inward if unable to point forward.

- Walk your left fingertips up the wall to create more length on the left side of your torso.

- Maintain full contact on the wall with your left hip and thigh by pressing into the mat with your right foot.

- Try to maintain length on both sides of your waist.

- Hold for 30 seconds to one minute and repeat on the other side.

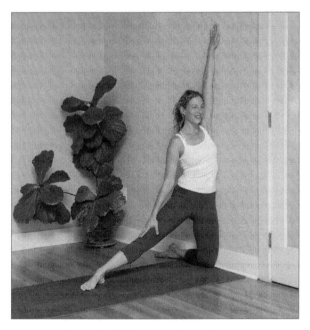

*Figure 4.13 Gate pose (Parighasana)*

At this stage of your therapeutic yoga journey, you have passed many important milestones. You have allowed yourself to move more deeply into the fine art of letting go. You have begun to develop, or at least to consider developing, personal qualities—including attitudes of non-violence, non-attachment, and discipline—that will serve both your yoga practice and your life. And you have learned postures (asana) that will create length and symmetry in your body. You are now ready to understand and practice the key principle involved in eliminating pain and discomfort in your spine: traction.

# CHAPTER 5

# Traction

In previous chapters, we discussed the first six steps in working with scoliosis:

1. Release muscular tension

2. Open your hips

3. Find your mountain pose

4. Strengthen the convex side

5. Lengthen the concave side

6. Create length and symmetry

In this chapter, we will move into the final physical technique, one that is beneficial for anyone with spinal conditions and especially those with scoliosis—traction. Most pain and dysfunction in the spine are due to compression, meaning a lack of space; something is being pinched and this results in a painful stimulus. What you may not know is that, even though your scoliosis may be causing symptoms such as sciatica, nerve root impingement, disc degeneration, or a bulging disc, to name just a few, it does not mean that you are destined to suffer. All you need to focus on is creating space between the vertebrae. Once the compression is relieved, the pain will disappear.

Consider the work presented by orthopedic physician Dr. John Sarno is his *Healing Back Pain: The Mind Body Connection* (1991). In this revolutionary book, he cites two research studies that explored the relationship between spinal abnormalities and back pain:

Between 1976 and 1980, two Israeli physicians, Dr. A. Magora and Dr. A. Schwartz, published four medical articles in the *Scandinavian Journal of Rehabilitation* in which they reported the results of studies they had done to determine whether certain spinal abnormalities caused back pain. Their method was to compare the X-rays of people with or without a history of back pain. If people with back pain had these abnormalities more commonly, one could presume that the abnormalities might be the cause of the pain.

They found no statistical difference in the incidence of degenerative osteoarthritis, transitional vertebra, spina bifida occulta, and spondylosis between the two groups. There was a small statistical significance for spondylolisthesis. In other words, once could not attribute back pain to these disorders, with the possible exception of spondylolisthesis.

A similar study was conducted by American radiologist Dr. C. A. Splithoff and published in the *Journal of the American Medical Association* in 1953. He compared the incidence of nine different abnormalities of the end of the spine in people with and without back pain. Again he found no statistical significance. (pp.131–132)

Several subsequent studies further confirmed Sarno's conclusions. These studies are indeed very encouraging; they can lead us to conclude that spinal abnormalities, including scoliosis, need not cause pain.

Traction helps create the decompression that leads to this pain-free outcome. But traction in Purna Yoga differs from most mechanical traction that you may have seen in physical therapy or chiropractic offices. In Purna Yoga, traction involves the careful, deliberate, and prolonged lengthening of a muscle or joint by submitting it to the *natural* force of gravity. Most other traction units exert an *external* pull on your spine, usually while you are lying down on your back. With the following techniques, you will use gravity and your own breath and awareness to accomplish lengthening in your own spine. You are in control.

Because of this, the body *learns* how to release the grip of the spinal muscles and allow the joints to move away from one another instead of being pulled apart by an aggressive outside force. When you work with gravity, the spine learns to let go bit by bit. Remember that the muscles around the spine become tight as a protective mechanism. The safer your body feels, the more the muscles will become soft and supple. Conversely, if there is a sudden force applied to the tension in the muscles, there is a risk that they will stretch briefly but will contract even harder moments later in response.

Again, visualize this principle as similar to a situation in which you are trying to get a toy out of a dog's mouth. If you pull at the toy, the dog will clamp down harder and pull back creating more resistance. If you simply distract the dog and soothe him by petting him, the dog will most likely soften and let go of his hold on the toy. Here is a simple truth: *You cannot force someone to let go.* The only way to encourage either physical or emotional release is to provide the right conditions, a sense of safety and security, which allow another person—or yourself—the opportunity to let go.

This is easier said than done, but the process of yoga will guide you towards letting go, albeit slowly, more and more each day, in body, mind, and soul.

So what is the best way to traction your spine when you have scoliosis?

A yoga wall would be your best bet and will yield the most improvement over time. There are alternatives to traction without installing a wall in your home, which I will explain in the following exercises. But the long-term benefits of installing a wall will outweigh the costs in no time. The following traction techniques are easy and safe to do and should be done three to five times a week for best results.

# Upright traction series

For the following standing traction series, you will need straps over a door (TRX or yoga straps can work) or a yoga wall with the two straps at the highest level. You can also hang from a trapeze-like bar. Monkey bars in a park can work to simulate this technique as well.

## *1. Standing traction*

- Hold onto the straps, with straps around your wrists, or onto the bar with the palms facing forward.

- Keep your back against the wall for support as you bend your knees and slide down the wall towards a seated position with your arms extended while holding onto the straps.

- Ensure that your shoulders are kept in joint and that the focus is on lengthening your torso between the armpit and the waist.

- Drop the weight of your pelvis downward, releasing your lower body towards the ground on every exhalation.

- Hold for ten deep breaths.

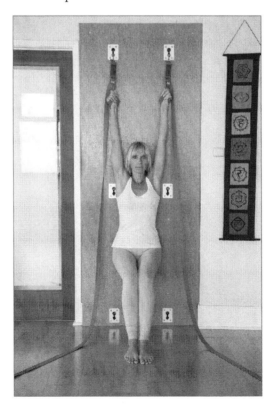

*Figure 5.1 Standing traction*

## 2. Pelvic rotation

- Repeat as in part 1, this time creating left spinal rotation by walking your feet towards the right. Keep your knees together for stability.

- Exhaling, drop the left side of your pelvis down towards the ground to facilitate traction with a twist. Imagine your pelvis moving further away from your rib cage with each breath.

- After a few deep breaths, walk your feet to the left and drop your right pelvis down.

- Hold for five to ten breaths.

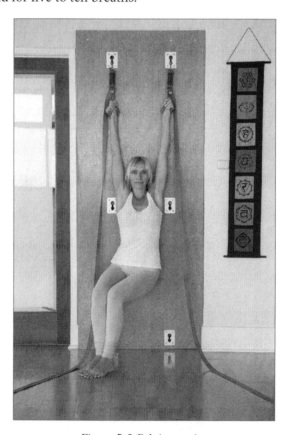

*Figure 5.2 Pelvic rotation*

# 3. Lateral flexion

*Note:* This posture is excellent for scoliosis, especially on the shortened side (concave side) of the curve, and should be practiced twice as much on the restricted side by individuals with an imbalance.

- Begin as in part 1 and walk both feet out to the side, stacking one foot directly on top of the bottom foot, creating a half-moon shape with the side body. Rest your spine against the wall for support.

- Sink your pelvis down towards the earth, keeping your shoulders in joint and lengthening the side of the waist and armpit area.

- Hold here for ten breaths as tolerated.

- If there is too much pressure on your hands and wrists, cross the top leg over the bottom and rest the foot on the floor (as in Figure 5.3 b.) for added support.

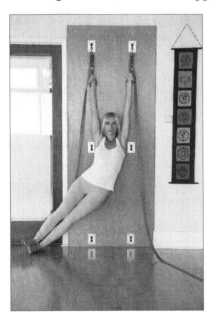 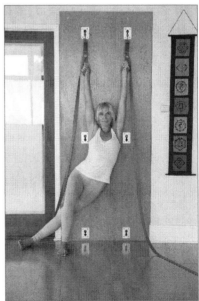

*Figure 5.3 a. Lateral flexion b. Lateral flexion (modified)*

# Hanging traction series

The next set of postures requires you to hang upside down, optimally with the use of a yoga wall. Effective as this position can be, it is not recommended if you have high blood pressure—even if you are on medication—a history of stroke or glaucoma, have had recent eye surgery, and during menstruation.

Hanging dog is one of the best ways to create traction in your lower back. Gravity assists the lengthening, while breath and awareness facilitate it. It is also fun! If you do not have a yoga wall, the posture can be done with a yoga strap on a door hinge or, preferably, with two yoga straps and a block over the top of a door.

## Set-up 1

- Loop two straps together making one longer strap.

- Place the end of the strap over a door hinge—in the opposite direction as the door would open—and feed the strap through, fastening it into a large circle.

- Adjust the strap so that it is roughly at the level of your hip creases.

- You will need to re-adjust as necessary so that your heels can touch the door, while the arms are outstretched on the ground, with the head three to six inches off the floor.

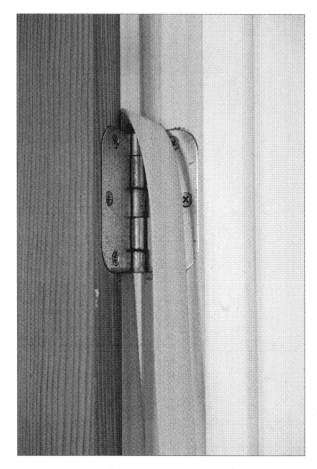

*Figure 5.4 Set-up 1 on a door hinge*

## Set-up 2

- Loop two straps together to make one big circle.

- Place a block in the circle and feed the block over the door, in the center, in the opposite direction of opening.

- Then close the door, testing the block to make sure that it is stable and can hold your weight on the strap.

- Adjust the strap so that it is roughly at the level of your hip creases.

- As above, you will need to re-adjust as necessary so that your heels can touch the door, while your arms are outstretched on the ground, with your head three to six inches off the floor.

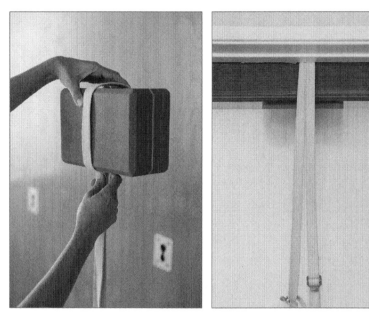

*Figure 5.5 Set-up 2 with a block in the center of the door (preferred)*

Now you should be set up in a supported downward-facing dog (Adho mukha svanasana) position with the heels up the door.

## *Hanging dog*

- Place your feet hip-distance wide and make sure that your feet are pointing straight ahead. Align the outer edges of your feet with the edges of your mat.

- Engage your thigh muscles as you extend your knees, feeling as if you are drawing your kneecaps up into the thighbones. Avoid "locking the knees" by pushing the knees back and rather focus on the lift in the frontal thighs towards your hip crease or groin area.

- Walk your hands out in front of you.

- Lengthen the shorter side of your curve by walking your hands away from the concavity. For example, if you have a right lumbar scoliosis, walk your hands to the right side to even out the curvature.

- Then add a gentle rotation of the rib cage to the opposite side. So, if you walk the hands to the right, twist to the left to normalize the rotational component of your curve.

- Take a deep inhalation.

- Exhaling, stretch out through your fingertips and lengthen the whole spine forward, beginning from your lower back/lumbar spine.

- Keep your lower belly slightly engaged to protect your lower back.

- Relax your head and neck.

- Hold here for one to two minutes.

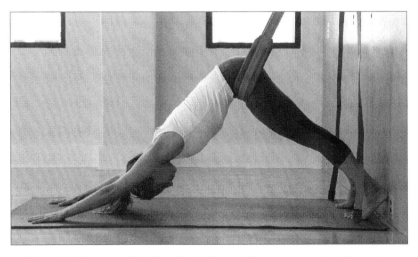

*Figure 5.6 Downward-facing dog (Adho mukha svanasana) with traction*

## Full traction on the pelvic swing

This technique is one of the most effective ways for you to release tension in your spinal muscles and to create length and symmetry. This pose is best practiced on a yoga wall for safety. *Practice this under the guidance of a trained Purna Yoga instructor before attempting on your own.*

- Be certain that the pelvic swing is at the level of your hip creases and not on the top of the thighs when coming into this position. If there is any pain in your thigh muscles, come down and reposition the swing so it rests higher up in your hip creases.

- Next, lean forward and place your hands on the floor and walk your feet up the wall so that your feet are slightly below hip level. Make sure your feet are roughly hip distance apart and your toes are pointing down towards the floor.

- Your head should be off the ground at least six inches.

- Rest the backs of your hands on the floor with the palms facing upward so that your upper back can remain relaxed.

*Note:* It is very helpful to have someone measure the distance from the crown of the head to the floor at the beginning and at the end of this exercise for reference. This measurement is a nice tool to show you how much length you have gained by hanging with the help of gravity and the breath.

- Take a deep inhalation, feeling the breath move into the lower back area.

- Exhaling, imagine the muscles between your vertebrae lengthening, increasing the intervertebral space.

- Release vertebra by vertebra with awareness, starting from your lower lumbar spine and moving up to the base of your neck.

- Hold for 10 to 20 breaths.

- When the release is complete, measure the distance from the crown of the head to the floor and notice if your spine gained some length!

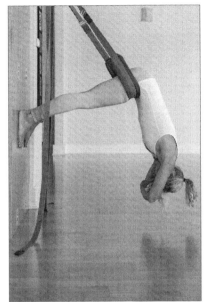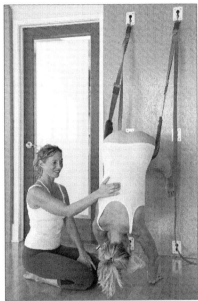

*Figure 5.7 Full traction on pelvic swing*

## Full traction with a side bend

- Begin by hanging in the pelvic swing as described above.

- Walk your hands to the side away from the concavity. For example, if you have a right lumbar scoliosis, walk your hands to the right. (Switch sides for a left scoliosis.)

- Place your right hand on top of the left hand to stabilize and lean your hips to the left.

- Breathe into the left (shortened) side of the body and feel your rib cage expanding with each inhalation.

- Hold for ten breaths.

- Practice twice as much on the shortened (concave) side for best results.

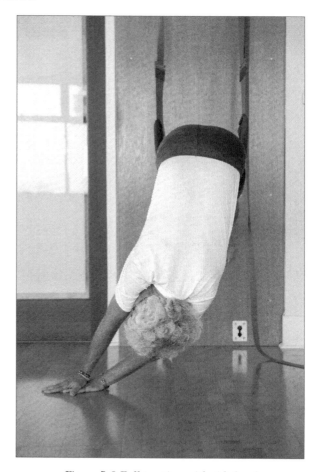

*Figure 5.8 Full traction with side bend*

With this chapter, we complete the physical postures, steps one through seven of the practices that will help you move towards normalizing your scoliosis. If you have also deepened your ability to practice the fine art of letting go and have continued to explore the personal ethics and attitudes embodied in the yamas and niyamas, you are well on your way to taking the final three steps of your journey. Yoga is the world's first mind–body medicine and these practices are derived from higher and more subtle aspects of the ancient science and philosophy of yoga. These three steps provide tools to help you explore the mind–body connection through the breath, mindfulness, and meditation.

# CHAPTER 6

# Mind–Body Tools

My yoga teacher, Aadil Palkhivala, tells a story about a day when he was travelling with his family and had to stop at a railroad track to wait for a train to pass by. At the railroad crossing, he got out of the car to watch the train. An older gentleman one car behind stepped out of his vehicle as well and walked over to Aadil. As the train approached, the man began to speak to my teacher. The noise of the train became louder and Aadil could not hear what the man was saying. He did not want to appear rude, however, so he nodded politely and smiled back at the man. Satisfied, the man returned to his car just as the train made its way towards its next stop.

About a half a mile down the road, Aadil came to a fork in the road and made a left turn as he was accustomed to. A few minutes later, he heard a loud "pop." He slowed down, realizing that his tire was flat. When he got out of the car, he noticed that broken glass all over the road had caused the puncture in the tire.

It was then that it occurred to him. The older gentleman at the train tracks had gotten out of his car to tell him that there had been an accident earlier and was warning him to avoid that particular road due to the broken glass from the wreck. However, since the noise of the train was so loud, he could not hear what the man was saying. Had he been able to hear the warning, Aadil may have been able to go a different route and avoid the flat tire altogether.

At the end of the story, my teacher paused. Then he said, "The older gentleman in the story represents your heart. The train represents the noise in your mind. The work of yoga is to quiet the noise in the mind so that you can listen to the soft whisper of your heart's longing."

While all the exercises presented in the preceding chapters can help you heal from chronic pain, tension, and complications due to your scoliosis, the real opportunity for change comes from within. It is my belief and my experience that true healing and well-being only occurs when you integrate mindfulness, meditation, and breathing into your life.

One of the most common problems resulting from scoliosis is negative self-image and a sense of having to "fight the curve" at all costs. This presents a situation in which you are constantly at odds with your own body. The key to letting go of physical tension is finding a way to be accepting of your body in its current state with an attitude of loving kindness. Maybe your spine is not perfectly straight, but who says that is the ideal? No reason can stop you from experiencing a full, happy, and pain-free life with scoliosis. In fact, you can even learn to love your curves.

Consider Danielle from Chapter 1. She went from being withdrawn, fearful, and disconnected from her body to loving her physical practice, welcoming touch, and being proud of her body no matter what. How did this happen? Was it the physical practice alone or was some other force at work?

After I approached her with genuine curiosity, Danielle told me that at the same time as she began working with me, she also started to work with a life coach. This coach helped her work with her belief system and judgments surrounding her scoliosis and helped her open up to a new way of being in her body and in her life. Coupled with the yoga practice, this awareness helped Danielle realize her inherent beauty and full, untapped potential. She made an active decision to embrace and love herself as she is, in this moment. This shift made all the difference. Being fully present with what is, with full acceptance and a sense of allowing, is exactly what a regular breathing and meditation practice can give you.

There are many paths and approaches towards being more embodied and aware. The next few exercises are suggestions that can help you begin to quiet the mind and connect to your heart while also focusing on correcting your scoliosis.

# Pranayama—Breath work

## *Lying over a bolster or blankets to prepare*

Lie lengthwise on a bolster with your chest supported on the bolster and your buttocks on the ground a few inches in front of the pillow. The bolster should be under your lower ribs, but not your lower back. The main intention is for your belly to move towards the legs and for the lungs to move towards your head, thereby freeing up the diaphragm to breathe more fully.

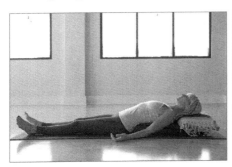
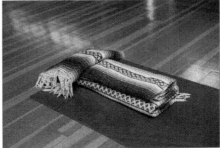

*Figure 6.1 Proper position for supine breath work: a. on bolster b. blanket set-up*

Place a blanket folded up neatly under your head so that the back of your head is supported and your chin is slightly tucked towards the center of your chest so that the gaze is towards the heart. Gaze internally towards the chest with soft eyes.

Rest your tongue on the bottom palate. In yoga, we keep the mouth closed and breathe in and out through the nostrils only. Keep your forehead, eyes, and eyelids soft and relaxed.

## *Belly breathing—Preparation for yogic breathing*

Start by placing your hands on your belly. On the inhalation, your belly should rise, as the diaphragm descends and pushes the abdominal contents forward. Conversely, your belly should fall on the exhalation, as the diaphragm recoils back up into the rib cage.

*In the beginning you may notice that you are breathing in the opposite manner; your belly may move inward on the inhalation and outward on the exhalation. Although this may feel natural to you, it is not the correct way to breathe. In fact, this pattern of breathing creates more tension in the neck muscles and also encourages a stress response. It may take a while to retrain your nervous system on how to breathe correctly. Be patient and it will feel more natural as you practice.*

Practice this breathing technique for five minutes in supine for a few weeks. Once you can do this comfortably, you can attempt the same exercise in a sitting position. Make sure you pay attention to the belly rising and falling on inhalation and exhalation respectively, and release any tension or activation in your neck muscles.

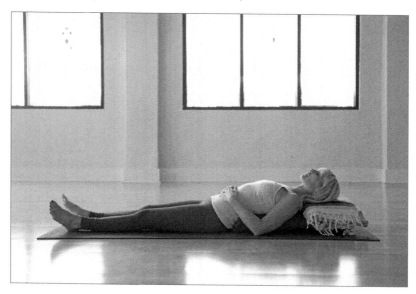

*Figure 6.2 Belly breathing*

## Three-part breathing in sitting

Sit up on a cushion or bolster so that the spine is in a neutral position. Place your hands on your lower ribs (one hand on each side) and inhale, filling up the lower lungs with breath. You may notice that one side of your rib cage is able to expand more than the other; this is common in individuals with scoliosis. Focus on trying to expand the restricted side by breathing into your hand more on that side. Repeat for 15 slow, deep breaths.

Then move the hands to the middle rib cage area, underneath your armpits, and take 15 breaths, filling up the middle lungs so that your ribs move out into your hands on each inhalation. Again, focus on breathing more into the restricted side by bringing your awareness to that area.

Finally, place your hands on the upper chest area close to the collarbones and complete 15 deep breaths, focusing on filling your upper lungs with breath.

If you find your mind wandering during this exercise, simply bring your attention back to the area on which you are focusing. Notice how you have the ability to direct the breath into different areas of your body with your awareness.

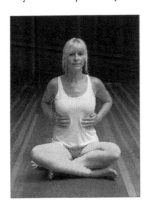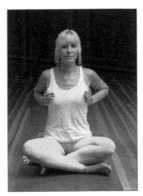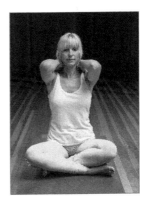

*Figure 6.3 Three-part breathing: a. lower lungs b. middle lungs c. upper lungs*

# Dhyana—Mindfulness and meditation

Meditation may be both the easiest and most difficult thing you will ever do in your life. It really is as simple as sitting, breathing, and continuously bringing your attention back to your breath. But somehow the ability to stop what we are doing and sit for even 10 to 15 minutes may seem impossible. If we all know that meditating can offer us more peace and calm in this unsettling world, why don't we do it more often? After all, it is completely free and available to us, anytime and anywhere.

If only it were that easy. Our minds are constantly at work trying to keep us busy being worried. Why? It really comes back to our built in survival instincts and our basic physiology. Because our nervous system is built for survival, like animals in the wild we are constantly on guard for danger and wired to worry about our safety and security. What makes us different from animals, however, is that we have the ability to retrain our brain so that our responses to external and internal stimuli are different from theirs. This does not happen by itself. In order to change thought patterns, reactions, and even our response to stress, we need to access the process of *neuroplasticity*. This attribute of the brain, sometimes known as brain plasticity, refers to the myriad of ways that neural pathways and synapses can change, actually reforming themselves, due to a person's changes in behavior, environment, neural processes, thinking, emotions, as well as from trauma and events that result in bodily injury. What this means is that direct *experience* can actually change the way our brain functions. The key to accomplishing this seemingly impossible task is through *repetition*. In order for our brain to learn how to process things and react differently, a new pathway needs to be created which requires a type of re-patterning that can only come from consistent practice. After time, because of the brain's neuroplasticity, the response will become automatic.

## Beginning meditation

We often think that meditation will quiet our minds so that we are free from thoughts and concerns. While that is sometimes one of the outcomes of a regular and consistent meditation practice, when you begin, you will notice that your mind will not stop jumping around from thought to thought. This is completely normal. The aim of meditation is to keep coming back to the present moment, over and over again. You will become the observer of your own thoughts and begin to notice how the mind is like a monkey jumping around from branch to branch. Over time, you will learn to watch the monkey with curiosity and amusement, but without attaching too much significance to each fleeting thought and emotion.

To begin meditation, find a comfortable seated position on a cushion or chair, making sure that the spine is straight and there is no tension in your back muscles. The knees should be lower than the hips to avoid slouching, as we want to maintain a natural lumbar curve. It may be helpful to sit with your back against a wall for support in the beginning until you build up enough strength to sit for longer periods of time.

Your goal will be to take ten quiet, even and deep breaths in and out through the nose. It sounds simple enough but keeping your mind focused enough to make it to ten is quite a feat! Observe your thoughts and the sensations that arise but do not place any meaning or significance on them. If you lose your count and notice your mind wandering, simply come back to your breath and focus on the quality of the inhalations and exhalations. Do this for ten breaths and keep redirecting your mind to the breath and the count, even if it is every single second. Try this simple technique every day, first thing in the morning. It will help you gain focus and a new perspective that will last all day long.

I often tell my clients that I think scoliosis is absolutely beautiful. When they look at me in disbelief I explain how it is a clear demonstration of the body's wisdom and innate desire to be in alignment. Scoliosis shows us that the body will do whatever it needs to so that we are as upright as possible and able to literally have our "heads on straight." What we can learn from this is that if we can remove some of the obstacles that prevent the spine from elongation—such as tightness or weakness in the muscles surrounding the spine as well as poor posture—the spine can find its way towards length without too much forcing. *We just need to provide the right conditions and the spine will straighten itself out.*

As with swimming in the open sea, the more we struggle and fight the current, the more tired and inefficient we become. The solution lies in the ability to let go and roll with the waves. Sometimes that requires more rest until the storm passes and sometimes it requires more effort to move ahead. But forcing is never the answer. Take a deep breath, and balance effort with ease. As you become more connected to what is happening in the ocean of your body, you will be able to use the tools presented here to help you live in peace and harmony with the currents of your spine and your life. There are so many things you can do to live a healthy, vibrant, and pain-free existence. Take the plunge today.

# Summary
PART III

## CHAPTER 7

# The Ten-Step Practice to Unwind Your Spine

### Step 1 Release muscular tension

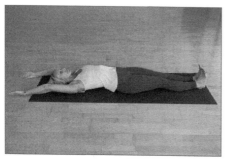

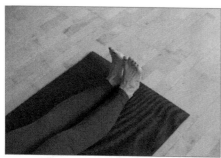

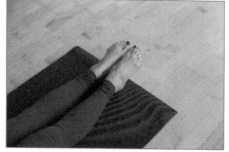

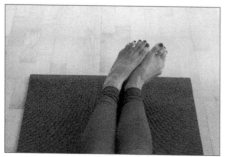

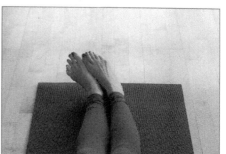

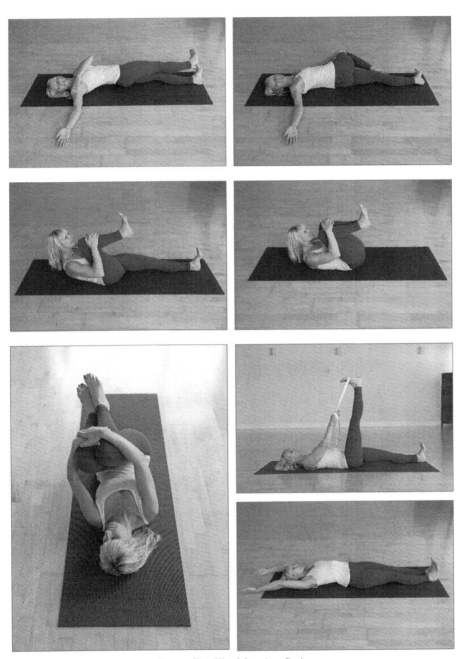

*Figure 7.1 The Morning Series*

# Step 2 Open your hips

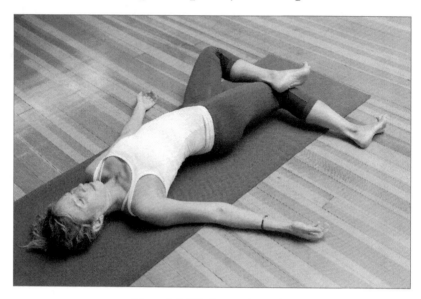

*Figure 7.2 Hip internal rotation*

# Step 3 Find your mountain pose

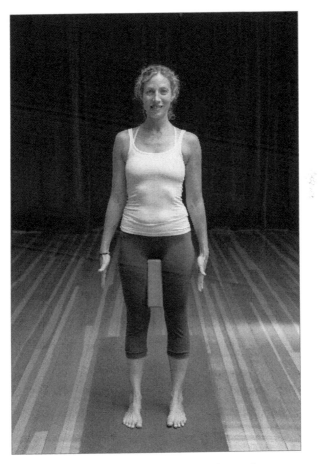

*Figure 7.3 Mountain pose (Tadasana)*

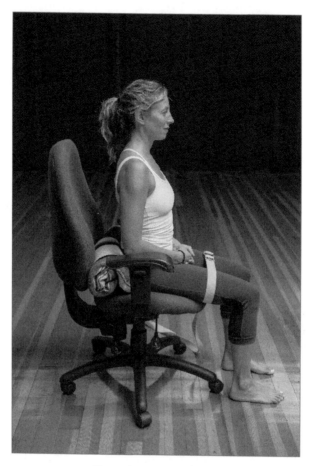

*Figure 7.4 Sitting posture*

# Step 4 Strengthen the convex side
## (practice with convex side down only)

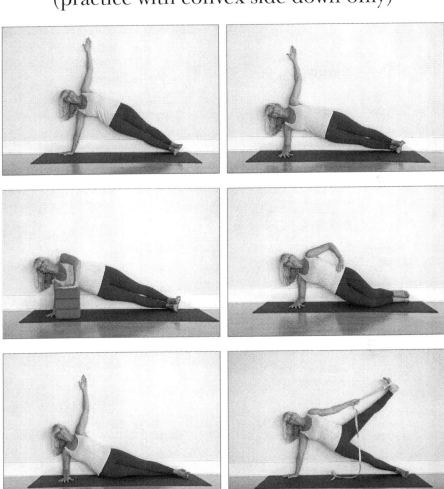

*Figure 7.5 Side plank variations*

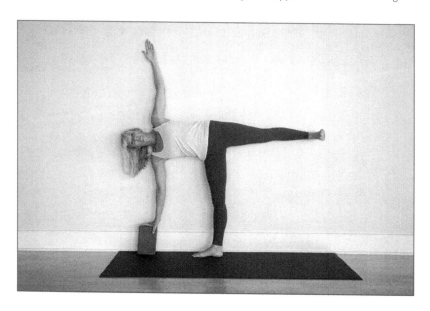

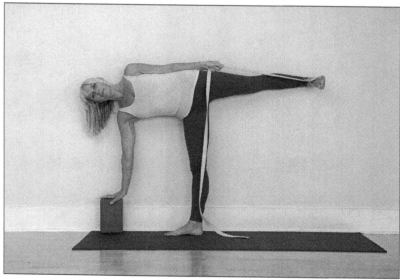

*Figure 7.6 Half-moon pose variations*

# Step 5 Lengthen the concave side
# (practice twice as much on concave side)

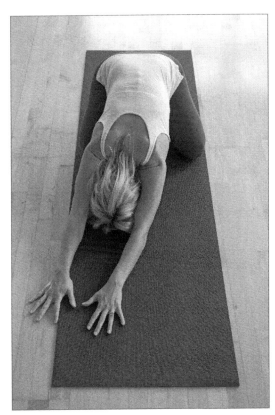

*Figure 7.7 Extended forward fold to one side*

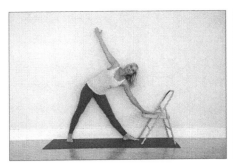 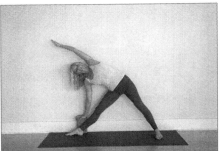

*Figure 7.8 Triangle pose (for right scoliosis): a. variation to lengthen the bottom side waist b. variation to lengthen the top side waist*

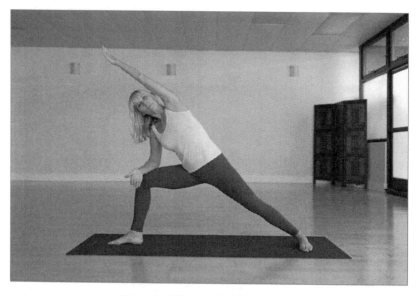

*Figure 7.9 Extended side angle pose*

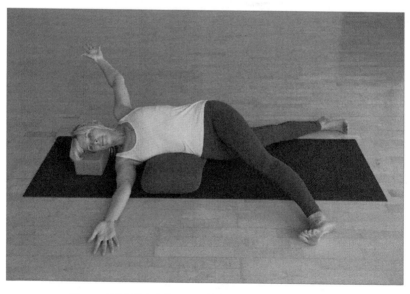

*Figure 7.10 Side-lying over bolster with trunk rotation*

## Step 6 Create length and symmetry

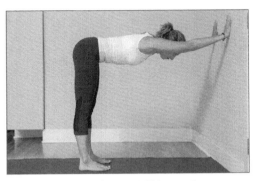

*Figure 7.11 Half-forward bend (Ardha uttanasana)*

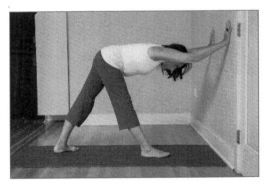

*Figure 7.12 Half-pyramid pose (Ardha parsvottanasana)*

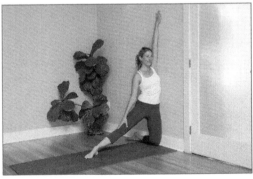

*Figure 7.13 Gate pose (Parighasana)*

# Step 7 Traction your spine

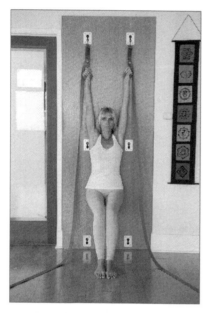 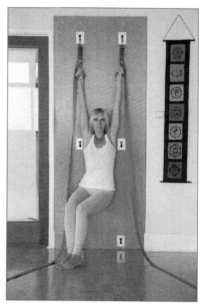

*Figure 7.14 Standing traction*         *Figure 7.15 Pelvic rotation*

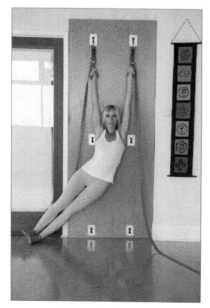 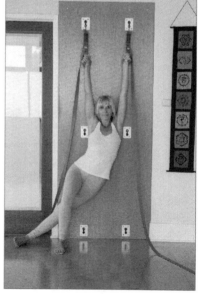

*Figure 7.16 a. Lateral flexion b. Lateral flexion (modified)*

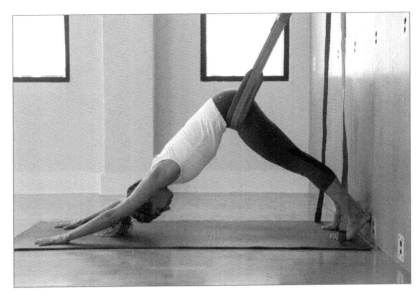

*Figure 7.17 Downward-facing dog with traction*

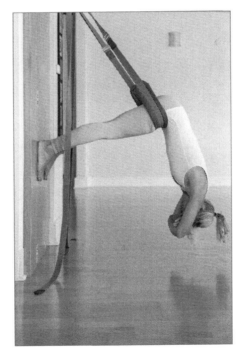

*Figure 7.18 Full traction on pelvic swing*

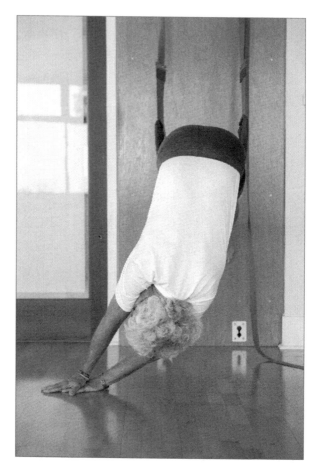

*Figure 7.19 Full traction with side bend*

# Step 8 Practice acceptance and surrender

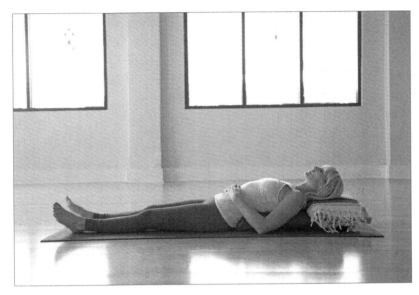

*Figure 7.20 Supported belly breathing*

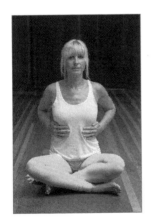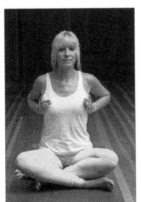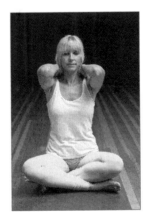

*Figure 7.21 Three-part breathing*

# Step 9 Quiet your mind

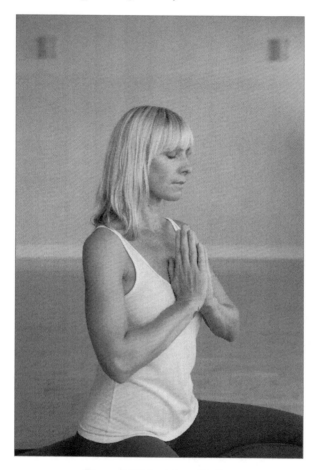

*Figure 7.22 Seated meditation*

# Step 10 Rest when you need it!

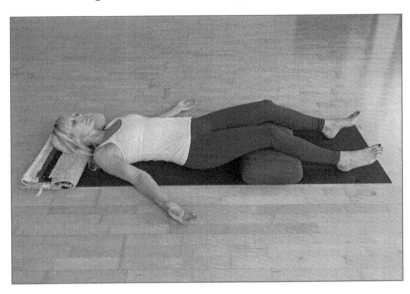

*Figure 7.23 Final relaxation pose (Savasana)*

# Bibliography

Browning-Miller, E. (2003) *Yoga for Scoliosis*. DVD and spiral-bound book, Shanti Productions.

Fishman, L., Groessl, E. J., and Sherman, K. J. (2014) "Serial case reporting yoga for idiopathic and degenerative scoliosis." *Global Advances in Health and Medicine 3*, 5, 16–21.

Mayo Clinic Staff (2015) *Complications of scoliosis*. Available at www.mayoclinic.org/diseases-conditions/scoliosis/basics/complications/con-20030140, accessed on April 6, 2016.

Monroe, M. (2012) *Yoga and Scoliosis: A Journey to Health and Healing*. New York, NY: Demos Medical Publishing.

Palkhivala, A. (2008) *Purna Yoga Teacher Training Manual*. Alive & Shine Center. *Purna Yoga™ founded by Aadil Palkhivala and Savitri*.

Sarno, J. (1991) *Healing Back Pain: The Mind Body Connection*. New York, NY: Warner Books/Hachette Book Group.

Satchitananda Sri Swami (trans.) (1978/2010) *The Yoga Sutras of Patanjali*. Buckingham, VA: Integral Yoga Publications.

Zaina, F., Romano, M., Knott, P., de Mauroy, J. C., *et al*. (2015) "Research quality in scoliosis conservative treatment: state of the art." *Scoliosis*. Available at www.ncbi.nlm.nih.gov/pmc/articles/PMC4537531, accessed on April 6, 2016.

Rachel Krentzman PT, E-RYT is the founder and director of Embody Physical Therapy and Yoga in San Diego, California, and is licensed as both a physical therapist and yoga therapist. As well as workshops and classes, Rachel offers teacher training in yoga therapy, particularly in the treatment of back problems. She lives in Israel.

Made in the USA
Middletown, DE
06 December 2021

54486139R00068